T0324926

Contemporary Challenges in Medical Education

Contemporary Challenges in Medical Education

From Theory to Practice

EDITED BY

ZAREEN ZAIDI, ERIC I. ROSENBERG,
AND REBECCA J. BEYTH

University of Florida Press

Gainesville

This book may be available in an electronic edition.

24 23 22 21 20 19   6 5 4 3 2 1

Library of Congress Cataloging-in-Publication Data
Names: Zaidi, Zareen, editor. | Rosenberg, Eric I., editor. | Beyth, Rebecca
 J., editor.
Title: Contemporary challenges in medical education : from theory to practice
 / edited by Zareen Zaidi, Eric I. Rosenberg, and Rebecca J. Beyth.
Description: Gainesville : University of Florida Press, 2019. | Includes
 bibliographical references and index.
Identifiers: LCCN 2018032357 | ISBN 9781683400745 (cloth : alk. paper)
Subjects: LCSH: Clinical medicine—Study and teaching. | Medicine—Study and
 teaching. | Medical education—Methods.
Classification: LCC R834 .C662 2019 | DDC 610.76—dc23
LC record available at https:// lccn.loc.gov/2018032357

UF PRESS

UNIVERSITY
OF FLORIDA

University of Florida Press
2046 NE Waldo Road
Suite 2100
Gainesville, FL 32609
http://upress.ufl.edu

Contents

Section I. Professional Development

Section II. Professionalism Issues

Section III. Implications for Teaching

Figures

Tables

Foreword

When the editors of this book, *Contemporary Challenges in Medical Education*, told me a bit about the purpose and story behind the book, I was instantly intrigued by the strong commitment to education signaled by such an endeavor. As I learned more about the genesis and evolution of this book project, I came to appreciate an additional commitment among the faculty members in the Division of General Internal Medicine at the University of Florida—a commitment to development of their scholarly community. For most clinician-educators, engagement in scholarship is expected but rarely granted protected time, resources, and mentorship. As such, it can be a lonely and frustrating part of academic life. This book project offers an inspiring example and refreshing change in approach. By carefully selecting author teams with varying degrees of experience in academic writing and assembling an editorial team to offer additional support to authors throughout the process, the book became a core activity of an emerging "community of practice" (Lave and Wenger 1991; Steinert 2010). By community of practice, I mean "a group of people who share a concern or passion for something they do and learn how to do it better as they interact regularly" (Wenger-Trayner, 2011). In my mind, this represents faculty development at its best.

The book produced through the work of this community of practice offers something quite unique to its readers. Its contents resonate with what Etienne and Beverly Wenger-Trayner describe as the "real body of knowledge" of a profession, namely, "the community of people who contribute to the continued vitality, application, and evolution of practice" (2011, p. 13). Books document some of this knowledge, but often just supply the sparks that ignite larger ideas and conversations. What gives knowledge power is subsequent uptake and application to practice. This book, *Contemporary Challenges in Medical Education: From Theory to Practice*, excites me because it reflects a dynamic, social learning process among an inspired, dedicated group of faculty at the University of Florida College of Medicine. The knowledge shared in its pages offers collective wisdom derived largely from practice (although grounded in existing literature) and is available to others to shape and implement in their own context.

This book is written primarily for practitioners—clinician-educators much like those who have written the chapters. The structure of each chapter lends itself to a variety of uses, from individual learning and improvement to collective faculty development. The chapters begin with objectives that can guide one's own learning or that can be used to facilitate faculty development sessions derived from the content. The subsequent content weaves together practical experience, discussed through vignettes and examples, with concise synthesis of existing literature and common conceptual frameworks applied to the topic. Each chapter concludes with set questions for future research as potential inspiration for those interested in delving more deeply into the topic and pursuing scholarship in the area.

The thirteen chapters are organized into three topical sections: I. Professional Development; II. Professionalism Issues; and III. Implications for Teaching. Each chapter brings to light common dilemmas encountered by clinician-educators, which I briefly touch upon below as a way of piquing the curiosity of readers and orienting those who may prefer to read chapters selectively rather than sequentially.

Chapters 1 through 5 in the section on professional development acknowledge human fallibility and provide readers with a rich compilation of resources related to well-being and resilience. Whether it is a time of transition from undergraduate education to graduate education or practice, or building and sustaining a career in academic medicine, the book can help readers gain insight by using the lens of "professional identity formation" and "graceful self-promotion."

The chapter "Focusing on Well-Being" describes a health care provider—Deborah—and her journey through academic medicine while facing personal and professional difficulties. The authors pull together literature from a variety of resources to examine factors influencing well-being and strategies to promote it, including easy-to-use autogenic training scripts and a guide to breathing exercises. This chapter is a concise resource for faculty on the topic of well-being with practical tools. The chapter on "Medical Error and Resilience" uses a clinical vignette to illustrate the toll of medical errors and fallibility on patients, clinicians, and the health care system, best practices for dealing with medical errors, and promotion of resilience as a countermeasure to burnout associated with medical errors. The chapter on "Attitude and Work Ethic" translates these abstract concepts into concrete factors backed by evidence to provide a framework of key factors influencing attitude and work ethics. The discussion on challenges to good attitudes and work ethics is useful for faculty in leadership positions.

The chapter "Professional Identity Formation" uses Jessica's case vignette to illustrate social identity theory. It differentiates between professionalism, virtue-based, and other behavior-based frameworks for professionalism in a way that makes these complex concepts accessible to the reader. In addition, the chapter explains how medical educators can use social identity theory during learners' transition periods, for example, medical school to residency training to a faculty position, specifically by building in time for reflection over the course of one's career, utilizing mentors, and obtaining feedback from others. The "Graceful Self-Promotion" chapter provides a much-needed resource for faculty endeavoring to successfully navigate their way in academia. The chapter addresses the fact that while it is important for faculty to ensure that their accomplishments receive appropriate recognition, they must deliver the message in a way that colleagues and superiors will not perceive as annoying, aggressive, or bragging. Health care professionals often find self-promotion to be challenging, and the chapter provides tips on how to do this gracefully and discusses cultural and gender issues that influence the process and consequently academic advancement.

Section II on professionalism has four chapters, which highlight professionalism issues in the context of power differentials, for example, microaggressions faced by minorities, pimping of learners, and impact of hierarchy within interprofessional teams.

The chapter "Teaching Women and Minorities" discusses microaggressions—what they are, the psychological impact, and how to counter them both at the individual and institutional level. The chapter on "Courage in Medicine" discusses the concept of *parrhesia*, which is a Foucauldian concept of "frankness in speaking the truth." The authors of this chapter discuss common ethical dilemmas that compel *parrhesia*, including witnessing unethical behavior, encountering conflicts being a team player

while honoring duty to the patient and dealing with "gallows or derogatory humor." They make recommendations for individuals and institutions to create environments that foster *parrhesia*.

The authors of the chapter "The Secret in the Care of the Learner"
interviewed faculty at the University of Florida who were repeatedly
recognized by students for excellence in teaching or humanistic skills to
identify strategies educators can use to create a positive educational experience. The authors summarize these strategies for readers in a table.
They also reviewed the literature on mistreatment, pimping, and Socratic
teaching and provide strategies for fostering and maintaining a safe learning environment in which learners feel unthreatened by questions posed
by educators. The "Teaching Humility and Avoiding Hierarchy" chapter
explores the differentials of hierarchy and power and how to find and
retain humility within medical education. It provides frameworks to understand the basis for power and practical steps to create awareness about
humility.

Section III brings forth issues that have implications for teaching, such as
how to discuss controversial topics with learners, how to teach in the era
of the electronic health record, and how to successfully instill and role-
model empathy for learners in busy clinical settings.

The chapter "A Framework for Discussing Controversial Topics in
Medical Education" uses case vignettes to model use of reflective rational
enquiry as a framework for discussing controversial topics that arise in
the clinical setting. It discusses approaches teachers can take when faced
with a controversial topic, including: denial that a topic is controversial,
using positions of power or privilege to teach toward a particular perspective, avoiding discussion of the topic, and trying to include different or
balanced perspectives in discussion. The chapter "Teaching in the Electronic Era" provides a framework for educators in this era of digital revo-
lution. It discusses teaching trainees how to document in the electronic
health record (EHR), the issues with EHR transparency, and addresses
ethical guidelines for social media use in medicine.

The differences between apprenticeship, mentorship, and role modeling are described in the chapter "Introspection about Role Modeling,"
with a summary of positive and negative attributes of role models that
will be handy for any educator. It brings up "role modeling consciousness," which is the awareness of one's role while interacting with trainees.

When we talk about work ethic and attitudes several abstract concepts come to mind. The "Teaching and Learning Empathy" chapter describes the importance of teaching empathy, discusses challenges to empathy, and provides strategies for empathy training.

This brief overview of the book offers just a glimpse of the vibrant landscape ahead. I encourage readers to fully appreciate the view from the field and the accompanying wisdom and insight so generously shared by what I have come to think of as an exemplary community of practice within Division of the General Internal Medicine at the University of Florida. I, and surely many others, am inspired by your commitment to education, scholarship, and, perhaps most of all, one another.

Bridget C. O'Brien, Ph.D.
Associate Professor, Department of Medicine
Educational Researcher, Center for Faculty Educators
School of Medicine
University of California, San Francisco

References

Lave, J., and Wenger, E. (1991). *Situated learning: Legitimate peripheral participation.* Cambridge, MA: Cambridge University Press.

Steinert, Y. (2010). Faculty development: From workshops to communities of practice. *Medical Teacher* 32(5): 425–428.

Wenger-Trayner, E., Fenton-O'Creevy, M., Hutchinson, S., Kubiak, C. and Wenger-Trayner, B. (2014). *Learning in landscapes of practice: Boundaries, identity, and knowledgeability in practice-based learning.* London and New York: Routledge.

Wenger-Trayner, E., and Wenger-Trayner, B. (2011). What is a community of practice? Available at: http://wenger-trayner.com/resources/what-is-a-community-of-practice (posted December 28). Last accessed February 24, 2018.

Preface and Acknowledgments

There is nothing to writing.
All you do is sit down at a typewriter and bleed.

Ernest Hemingway

We begin with the story of how this book came to be. In 2015, our Division of General Internal Medicine's strategic planning retreat resulted in a commitment to improve the quality of ambulatory medicine training for our learners. The faculty conceived a "Clinician Educator's Manual" to disseminate the resources many had created for teaching. However, this rapidly evolved into a more ambitious division-wide "book project." The book specifically addresses gaps in the medical education literature where there had been controversy and vigorous debate, or where faculty had consistently asked for assistance. The chapters were authored by well-respected faculty teachers and faculty experienced in medical education research. A select number of faculty were invited as authors from outside the institution (nationally and internationally) on some chapters. The faculty authors are mainly clinician-educators with several in leadership roles in medical education. Our belief is that their input as faculty from the "field" providing real-life experiences moves this collection of text from being just ivory-tower concepts to being immediately applicable to health profession educators. We requested all authors to clearly state "conceptual frameworks" to inform readers about the theories they used to build the narrative of the chapters and avoid abstract discussions of topics. The vignettes at the start of the chapters are from the faculty's own real-life experiences dealing with medical students, residents, peers, and other health care professionals.

The Division of General Internal Medicine assisted the process in several ways, including holding workshops focused on methods to overcome procrastination and strategies for collaborative writing projects. The division provided resources such as dedicated academic time for faculty to develop their topics, consult with a librarian, and undertake literature reviews. Assistance was provided on using a reference management tool, using a conceptual framework, and dealing with typical editorial concerns.

The College of Medicine librarian provided support to the project by undertaking literature reviews on each of the topics and creating folders on a shared institutional drive. To further aid the faculty, our librarian imported these references into a reference manager, RefWorks, so that our faculty could "cite as they write." Gwen Martin, our editorial assistant, meticulously reviewed every iteration of the chapters. The Division Chief for General Internal Medicine (one of the editors), the Chair of the Department of Medicine, and the Deans at the College of Medicine extended administrative support and, importantly, moral support, cheering the team on.

The collaborative writing process had several ripple effects at our institution, including an increased awareness of institutional academic support structures and increased interactions between faculty working at different clinical sites in the city and faculty outside our institution. We invite our readers to engage in further conversations on topics covered in this book through the research questions provided at the end of every chapter.

Finally, we'd like to share a few tips for designing and bringing large collaborative projects such as this to fruition:

1. Ensure you have a clearly defined document that lays out "unifying features" for all chapters, including word count, font, line spacing, chapter structure, common elements and reference format.
2. Consider how you plan to "nurture writing relationships." Team-building exercises and discussion of roles of authors are important steps.
3. Discuss the writing process of the book, including the natural editing processes; for example, how to handle and respond to major or minor revisions.
4. Consider opportunities for faculty development related to academic writing over an extended period; this may provide faculty with opportunities to raise issues they are encountering.

As Helen Keller famously said, "Alone we can do so little, together we can do so much." Although at times faculty authors did likely feel like they were "bleeding" at the proverbial typewriter, overall, as we drew to a completion of the book, we could see firsthand the power of the writing groups. The authors drew strength from each other and were resilient to critiques from the editors. We would like to thank them for taking a leap of faith with this project, for their dedication, for the countless hours they have given to preparing the manuscript, and for entrusting us with their hard work. During the process, we would not have been successful if it were not for many other individuals. We would like to take the opportunity to offer them our sincerest appreciation for being the wind beneath our wings:

Maureen Novak, M.D.—Associate Dean, Medical Education

Robert Hromas, M.D.—Former Chairman, Department of Medicine

Meredith Babb—Director, University Press of Florida

Gwen Martin—Line Editor at Gwen's Red Pen

Hannah Norton—Associate University Librarian, Health Science Center Libraries

Shaima Coffey—Assistant Director, Healthcare Administration, Division of General Internal Medicine

Marilyn Nehring—Administrative Support Assistant II, Division of General Internal Medicine

Samantha Gulick—Administrative Support Assistant II, Division of General Internal Medicine

*   *   *

To my parents to whom I am grateful for inspiring me to reach higher and for instilling resilience; to my husband and boys for their unwavering support and encouragement through thick and thin.—Zareen Zaidi

With grateful thanks to Morris and Cristina Rosenberg, the first and most important teachers in my life.—Eric Rosenberg

To all learners and teachers who strive on a daily basis for self-improvement. To my family who keep me grounded and give me strength for all I do.—Rebecca Beyth

SECTION I

Professional Development

1

Focusing on Well-Being

IRENE M. ESTORES AND MARGARET C. LO[1]

Festina lente—Make haste slowly.
Latin translation of Classical Greek adage

We propose a conceptual framework for how institutions, educators, and learners can promote well-being. We provide personal strategies for mindfulness training, relaxation techniques, appreciative inquiry, narrative medicine, and positive psychology. We review the Liaison Committee on Medical Education (LCME) and the Accreditation Council for Graduate Medical Education (ACGME) initiatives to promote a culture of well-being in health systems, as well as individual and organizational initiatives.

Objectives

Describe factors that influence the well-being of health profession educators and learners.

Provide a framework to promote personal strategies to enhance well-being among learners.

Provide resources for implementation and research on wellness.

Deborah is a 34-year-old emergency medicine physician facing a professional and personal crossroads. As a child, she had a keen interest in science, and her parents encouraged and praised her aspirations. Despite her best effort, she did not graduate at the top of her class. She considered this a major failure, and vowed to intensify and focus her efforts on academic work in the future.

---

1 Irene M. Estores, M.D., University of Florida College of Medicine, Gainesville, FL.
Margaret C. Lo, M.D., F.A.C.P., University of Florida College of Medicine, Gainesville, FL.

Deborah was unsuccessful at her first attempt to get into medical school. Once admitted, she adjusted well to the rigors of medical school until her second year when her father died suddenly. Her classmates noticed she now preferred to study alone and was losing weight. She felt depressed, but feared disclosing this. She told herself she had no time to spare for counseling or therapy. She struggled quietly with her depression, graduated from medical school, completed an emergency medicine residency, and married.

Deborah thought her professional and personal life was on track. Then, a medical error resulted in a medical malpractice lawsuit. Despite the case's eventual resolution, she remained anxious, and worried constantly about making a medical error. Her colleagues noticed she was impatient and irritable. She questioned her decision to be a physician, as well as the value of her work. Several colleagues offered to cover extra shifts so she could take an extended vacation. Her husband was also worried and encouraged her to consider a career change. She recognized she had burnout, and sought help.

Factors That Influence Well-Being

Well-being is an internal state characterized by a predominance of positive emotions (contentment, happiness, a sense of fulfillment) and positive functioning (Diener 2000). It has become a public health outcome due to its association with self-perceived health, healthy behaviors, and productivity (CDC 2016). Determinants of well-being include genetics, personality, gender, age, and external factors such as income, work, and relationships (Nes et al. 2006). Heritability studies suggest that genetics may determine positive emotions, but they also recognize the role of environmental factors (Nes et al. 2006). Well-being is positively associated with the personality traits of optimism, high self-esteem, and extroversion while neuroticism is negatively associated with it (Diener 2000).

Low self-esteem, obsessive worry, social anxiety, intolerance of uncertainty, and fear of personal inadequacy and failure impact well-being negatively (McCranie and Brandsma 1989; Bovier and Perneger 2007; Gerrity et al. 1990). Most health care professionals, like Deborah, have personality traits predating their education that act as endogenous stressors or resilience facilitators (Benbassat et al. 2011).

Deborah is experiencing multiple components of burnout:

Emotional fatigue resulting in loss of passion for medicine
Depersonalization leading to cynicism and disinterest at the workplace
An overwhelming sense of personal and professional ineffectiveness (Maslach et al. 1996; Thomas 2004).

Personal, situational, and professional stressors all contribute negatively to well-being.

Personal factors

Deborah's case illustrates several personal factors negatively affecting well-being. These are: financial stress from educational indebtedness (Collier et al. 2002; Sargent et al. 2004; McNeeley et al. 2013); inadequate coping skills, especially anxious-avoidance or denial leading to self-doubt and self-criticism (Bittner et al. 2011; Firth-Cozens 2001); and a history of psychiatric disorder, especially depression (Campbell et al. 2010; Ford and Wentz 1984; Hirschfeld and Klerman 1979). Also negatively impacting well-being are social isolation—for example, moving to a new town, lacking peer support or relationships, or having little to no family engagement (Rutherford and Oda 2014); negligence in self-care and leisure activities; and antisocial, avoidant, or dependent personality disorder (Lemkau et al. 1988; Purdy et al. 1987). Other factors negatively associated with well-being include youth, single marital status, and childlessness (Collier et al. 2002; Eneroth et al. 2014; Kimo Takayesu et al. 2014; Martini et al. 2004; Sargent et al. 2004; Shanafelt et al. 2002). The impact of gender and ethnicity on resident well-being remains ambiguous (Ishak et al. 2009; Prins et al. 2007; Ripp et al. 2011; Thomas 2004).

Situational factors

A supportive learning environment with esprit de corps allows protective measures to take place (Aach et al. 1988; Dyrbye and Shanafelt 2016; Eckleberry-Hunt et al. 2009; Ishak et al. 2009; Prins et al. 2007; Rutherford and Oda 2014; Satterfield and Becerra 2010; Thomas 2004). A malignant learning environment—that is, where there is hostility among peers or faculty, program indifference to residents' suggestions, or lack of feedback on self-performance—can worsen physician burnout (Kimo Takayesu et al. 2014; Ripp et al. 2011; Sargent et al. 2004). Other situational factors negatively associated with well-being are: excessive or inappropriate administrative responsibilities; insufficient resources or ancillary support, including lack of allied health personnel; excessive or heavy time demands or duty hours leading to work exhaustion and sleep deprivation; and overwhelming or inadequate workload, including patient census or ward call volume (Sargent et al. 2004).

Professional factors

Professional factors can have a positive or negative impact on physician well-being (Aach et al. 1988; Dyrbye and Shanafelt 2016; Eckleberry-Hunt et al. 2009; Ishak et al. 2009; Prins et al. 2007; Rutherford and Oda 2014; Satterfield and Becerra 2010; Thomas 2004; Wallace, Lemaire, and Ghali 2009). Some factors are essential to develop medical knowledge and clinical skills, and to engender confidence and competency in medicine. For example, the long-standing culture of graduated resident autonomy and responsibility for patient care, teaching, supervision, and leadership can create resilience in the face of personal adversity.

Other professional risk factors are ambiguous roles and responsibilities in patient care (Kimo Takayesu et al. 2014), a lack of independence or control over work schedule or patient care (Kimo Takayesu et al. 2014; Ripp et al. 2011; Zwack and Schweitzer 2013), and excessive supervisory or teaching responsibilities of junior learners. Overwhelming exposure to difficult, complex patients or clinical pathology, lack of career mentoring and planning, and fear of patient safety errors or medical litigation negatively affect physician well-being (Levin et al. 2007).

Conceptual Framework

We present a framework demonstrating the intersection of personal practices, institution-sponsored programs, and national initiatives (Figure 1) illustrating how institutions and learners can promote well-being.

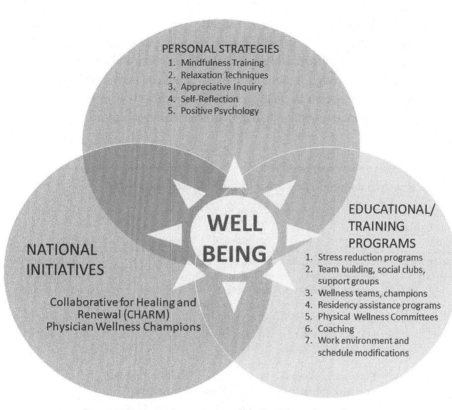

Figure 1. Strategies to promote well-being. Figure by authors.

Personal Strategies

Mindfulness training

Mindfulness is a state of awareness achieved by nonjudgmentally paying attention in the present moment (Paulson et al. 2013). Mindfulness is a trait that develops from consistent formal mindfulness-meditation practice and use in daily life (Kiken et al. 2015). Several health professional curricula incorporate mindfulness. These include the Mindfulness Based Stress Reduction program (MBSR), which is a mind-body skills training program; the Embodied Health program of yoga and meditation with a neuroscience didactic component; and an online, peer-facilitated program (Rosenzweig et al. 2003; Erogul et al. 2014; Greeson et al. 2015;

Maclaughlin et al. 2011; Kraemer et al. 2016; Bond et al. 2013; Kemper and Yun 2014). Participants noted improvements in perceived stress, mood, stress biomarkers, distress tolerance, self-compassion, and affect (Table 1). Although these programs are feasible and beneficial in promoting mindfulness and relaxation in medical school curricula, their impact on academic performance and empathy in clinical settings is unknown.

Table 1. Research on mind-body programs in U.S. medical schools

First Author and Publication Date	Study Design	Intervention	Outcome Measures	Results
Rosenzweig et al. (2003)	Prospective nonrandomized, cohort-controlled study N=140 (intervention) N=162 (controls) 1st year MS.	10-wk MBSR course as elective control: didactic course on CAM.	POMS	Significant improvement in POMS scores post-MBSR intervention.
Maclaughlin et al. (2011)	Prospective, nonrandomized, cohort-controlled study N=24 (intervention), N=22 (control) 1st year MS.	11-wk Mind Body Skills program as elective control: no intervention.	Salivary cortisol, DHEA testosterone, and IgA levels.	
Bond et al. (2013)	Prospective pre- and postintervention study.	11-week Embodied Health elective N=27.	JSE PSS SRQ SCS Qualitative data from postcourse essays.	Decreases in perceived stress, improvement of self-regulation, self-compassion, empathy.
Erogul et al. (2014)	Prospective, randomized, cohort-controlled trial, N=58 1st year MS.	Intervention: 8-week MBSR. Control: no intervention.	PSS BRS SCS Measured postintervention, and after 6 months.	Improvements in perceived stress and self-compassion seen postintervention and after 6 months. Improvement in resilience postintervention.

First Author and Publication Date	Study Design	Intervention	Outcome Measures	Results
Greeson et al. (2015)	Prospective, pre- and postintervention study N=44 MD, and MD-Ph.D. students (1st, 2nd, 3rd and 4th year MS).	4-week Mind-Body Skills workshop (abbreviated version of 11-week program) N=44.	CAMS-R PSS-10 Qualitative data on perceived value of the workshop.	Decreases in perceived stress and improvements in mindfulness.
Kemper and Yun (2014)	MD students.	8-week online training program, peer-facilitated 7 started, 4 completed.	PSS-10 CAMS-R BRS SCS CCCS SEQ	Changes in frequency of meditation practice.
Kraemer et al. (2016)	Prospective, cohort-controlled, nonrandomized 1st and 2nd year MS.	11-week MBS training course offered as elective.	DTS CAMS PSS-10 PANAS Qualitative data	Improvement in distress tolerance.

Compiled by authors.
Abbreviations:
BRS—Brief Resilience Scale
CAM—Complementary and Alternative Medicine
CAMS-R—Cognitive and Affective Mindfulness Scale, Revised
CCCS—Calm, Compassionate Care Confidence Scale
DHEA—Dehydroepiandrostenedione
DTS—Distress Tolerance Scale
IgA—Immunoglobulin A
JSE—Jefferson Scale of Empathy
MBSR—Mindfulness Based Stress Reduction
MD—Medical Doctor
MS—medical student
PANAS—Positive and Negative Affect Scale
Ph.D.—Doctorate of Philosophy
POMS—Profile of Mood States
PSS—Perceived Stress Scale
PSS-10—Perceived Stress Scale–10
SCS—Self-Compassion Scale
SEQ—Self-efficacy in providing nondrug care to relieve symptoms
SRQ—Self-Regulation Questionnaire

Relaxation techniques

Relaxation techniques activate the body's innate relaxation response through slow deep breathing, muscle tension reduction, or suggestions evoking a state of tranquility. It results in significant reductions in distractive and ruminative behaviors, situational anxiety, and other mood disturbances (Jain et al. 2007; McCray et al. 2008; Wild et al. 2014). A recent meta-analysis (Conley et al. 2015) found relaxation training was the most beneficial skills-based intervention strategy (mean effect size [mES]=0.55, confidence interval [CI]=0.41–0.68), proceeded by mindfulness (mES=0.34, CI=0.19–0.49) and cognitive behavioral therapy (mES=0.49, CI=0.40–0.58), meditation exercises (mES=0.25, CI=0.02–0.53), and finally psychoeducational training (mES=0.13, CI=0.06–0.21). The critical component of the intervention was supervised practice during the skills-based training (Conley et al. 2015).

Four major relaxation techniques exist to cope with stress.

Autogenic training utilizes self-suggestion to produce physical relaxation (Textbox 1) (Schultz and Luthe 1959).

Textbox 1. Sample autogenic training script

- Sit comfortably with back supported, feet flat on the floor, arms resting on the thighs.
- Close your eyes and notice the pattern and rhythm of the breath without trying to control the rate or rhythm of the breath.
- Imagine the "in and out" movement of the breath as a wave moving in and out on the beach, bringing to mind the sensation of warmth.
- Repeat the following statements quietly about three to six times:
  - My hands are heavy and warm; I am at peace.
  - My legs are heavy and warm; I am at peace.
  - My abdomen radiates warmth; I am at peace.
  - My heartbeat is strong and steady; I am at peace.
  - My breath is smooth and effortless; I am at peace.
  - My forehead is cool and comfortable; I am at peace.
  - My body balances itself perfectly; I am at peace.

The exercise typically takes about 10 minutes to complete.

Courtesy of Nancy Haraduk, Georgetown School of Medicine's Mind Body Skills Program (permission granted by Nancy Harazduk via email communication, March 24, 2017).

Guided visualization uses a trained therapist, coach, or a prerecorded CD prompting a series of mental images for a visual journey to a tranquil, peaceful place engaging the five senses. Guided visualization is also used to attain professional goals, for example, visualizing every step of a morning report presentation in advance to bolster self-confidence when speaking to a large group.

Progressive muscle relaxation slowly and progressively tenses and relaxes each individual muscle group starting with the toes and moving to the head. The learner repeats a sequence of 5 seconds for tension, and 30 seconds for relaxation.

Breathing techniques promote deep relaxation and a clear state of mind via abdominal or diaphragmatic breathing and 4-7-8 Breathing (Textboxes 2 and 3).

Textbox 2. Abdominal breathing exercise

- Place one hand on the chest and the other on the abdomen.
- Inhale with a slow, deep breath through the nose, ensuring the diaphragm (not the chest) fully inflates the lung and the abdomen is pushing against the hand.
- Exhale slowly through the mouth.
- Repeat for 6 to 10 slow, deep breaths per minute for 10 minutes each day.

Courtesy of Nancy Haraduk, Georgetown School of Medicine's Mind Body Skills Program (permission granted by Nancy Harazduk via email communication, March 24, 2017).

Textbox 3. The 4-7-8 relaxation breathing exercise

- Either lie down flat on your back or sit comfortably with back straight up.
- Place the tip of the tongue against the back of the two upper front teeth, and keep it there through the entire exercise.
- Begin the exercise by closing the mouth and inhaling quietly through the nose to a mental count of 4.
- Hold breath for a mental count of 7.
- Exhale completely and loudly with a whoosh sound through the mouth, to a mental count of 8.
- This is one complete breath. Repeat this cycle of 4-7-8 breathing 3 more times for 4 breaths.
- Practice this exercise at least 2 times a day but no more than 4 complete breaths at one time in the initial month of practice.

Courtesy of Dr. Andrew Weil, https://www.drweil.com.

Appreciative Inquiry

The original application of Appreciative Inquiry was to create positive change in organizations and social systems (Bushe 1995). The process centers on a 4-D (Discovery, Dream, Design, Destiny) cycle and posits that change is best effected by identifying strengths and best practices, rather than by focusing on the problem. Components of Appreciative Inquiry were adapted to reduce psychological distress and burnout in physicians (Krasner et al. 2009), and to coach trainees (Palamara et al. 2015; Daskivich et al. 2015) (see Appendix).

Narrative medicine

Narrative medicine upholds the three fundamental tenets of attention, representation, and affiliation to cultivate skills of listening, empathizing, reflecting, and crafting stories to connect with patients (Charon 2007). It closes the chasm between physicians and patients through meaningful patient engagement, unconditional patient-physician bonds, insight into one's own internal feelings, and acceptance of patients' perspectives (Greenhalgh and Hurwitz 1999; Charon 2001, 2007).

Educational pedagogies in narrative-based medicine curricula include reflective-writing portfolios, focus support group sessions, literature discussion group sessions, and Balint groups (de Vibe et al. 2013; Pololi and Frankel 2001; Wald 2015; Gardiner et al. 2015; Winkel et al. 2010; Bar-Sela et al. 2012; Novack et al. 1997). Balint group activities focusing on patient-centered management and strong patient-doctor relationships are the most promising intervention in preventing physician burnout and reducing anxiety or work-related exhaustion. Modest improvements in learners' empathy and job-related stress occurred during the intervention, but benefits diminished when the intervention ended (Fares et al. 2016; Novack et al. 1999; Romani and Ashkar 2014; Zwack and Schweitzer 2013).

Educational and clinical practices use four major categories of narratives (Kalitzkus and Matthiessen 2009):

Patient Stories: patients write their personal medical experiences and emotional turmoil in a classic illness-narrative. They reflect on lessons learned, copings skills used, and personal growth obtained from their experiences. The sharing of reflections helps physicians connect with their patients suffering.

Physicians' Stories: doctors detail the life and experiences of caring for the ill. These reflections expose physicians' vulnerabilities and humanize the medical process. It also promotes bonding and connectedness when shared with others.

Narratives about Physician-Patient Encounters: patients detail their illness by reflecting on the interplay between their illness and their physician as diagnosticians and healers. They share their stories with physicians who can exert a positive or negative influence on these narratives, although the degree of influence is unclear.

Metanarratives: these are global stories on the sociocultural aspects of the human body in relationship to illness and health. They reflect on medical history or the interconnection between experiences related to understanding illness and the ailing human body (Kalitzkus and Matthiessen 2009; Morris 1993).

Positive psychology

Cultivation of positive emotions is another means to counteract the negative emotions learners' experience. It focuses on strengths as the means to improve outcomes and is based on the hypothesis that individuals create a protective buffer during stressful times (Seligman et al. 2005). Positive psychology offers simple self-administered interventions, including the Three Good Things exercise, gratitude letters, the Best Possible Self exercise, and PERMA (Positive Emotion, Engagement, Relationships, Meaning, Accomplishment; see Appendix). In the Three Good Things exercise, learners reflect on three things that went well and their causes daily for one week. Variations include three things accomplished, three things grateful for, or three strength-building things per day. In gratitude letters, learners identify one individual for whom they are grateful and write an intimate letter of gratitude to them. There is no obligation to send or share the letter; they reflect on how they felt expressing gratitude. College undergraduates improved their positive affect after four weeks of using these interventions (Sheldon and Lyubomirsky 2006).

A Culture of Well-Being in Health Systems

Initiatives by LCME and ACGME

The Liaison Committee on Medical Education (LCME) and the Accreditation Council for Graduate Medical Education (ACGME) issued accreditation standards to implement well-being promotion, fatigue management, and burnout prevention for trainees, which included the ongoing assessment of learner burnout, easy access to confidential counseling, and resident duty hour restrictions (Daskivich et al. 2015). Although the regulations acknowledge the need to cultivate a culture of well-being in the medical education community, they offer little guidance on the most effective process or programs to accomplish this goal.

Among medical trainees, a systematic review identified five interventions demonstrating benefits in stress reduction and well-being promotion (Shapiro, Shapiro, and Schwartz 2000). Interventions included relaxation training, mindfulness meditation, cognitive behavioral therapy, narrative medicine, support group sessions, and personal or team-building social activities (Aach et al. 1988; Cedfeldt et al. 2015; Epstein and Krasner 2013; Hochberg et al. 2013; Joules et al. 2014; Longenecker et al. 2012; Satterfield and Becerra 2010; Veldenz et al. 2003; West et al. 2014; Zwack and Schweitzer 2013). Others noted benefits from peer mentorship to reduce stress, cultivate collegiality, or reaffirm career happiness (Eckleberry-Hunt et al. 2009; Ramanan et al. 2006). Programs fully integrated across the medical education continuum have had some success (Dabrow et al. 2006).

The seven essential recommendations for a national academic policy on resident well-being by the ACGME Council of Review Committee Residents (Daskivich et al. 2015) are:

Increase awareness and destigmatize anxiety and depression.

Introduce formal institutional processes to identify and address trainees' mental health issues.

Organize faculty development on well-being strategies.

Foster a supportive collegial institutional culture through regularly scheduled well-being activities.

Establish ongoing monitoring of residents for signs of burnout or mental health issues.

Cultivate close mentorship by faculty or senior colleagues.

Offer convenient, free access to mental health services with expanded hours.

The University of San Diego School of Medicine and the U.S. Air Force offer well-cited, multiprong strategies incorporating anonymous burnout screening, confidential treatment of mental illness, and formal skills-building curricula on well-being strategies, mental health education, and stress management for physicians at all stages (Moutier et al. 2012; Sheikhmoonesi and Zarghami 2014; Goldman et al. 2015; Reynolds and Clayton 2009). Learners have protected time for participation. The top-down approach of these programs is key to their success (Ramanan et al. 2006).

Individual and organizational initiatives

Individual-focused programs use cognitive and/or behavioral interventions to improve physicians' work performance and career satisfaction. Training includes adaptive coping skills, communication skills, psychotherapy, focus support groups, mentorship, and relaxation or mindfulness techniques (Awa et al. 2010; Schrijver 2016; Shanafelt 2009; West et al. 2014). The majority of these show significant reductions in burnout and in risk factors against well-being (Awa et al. 2010); however, they do not last beyond six months.

Organization-focused programs focus on practice redesign, job restructuring, or leadership innovations (Awa et al. 2010; Dunn et al. 2007; Schrijver 2016). They aim to increase job autonomy, decrease work demands, improve practice conditions, empower physicians, or promote physician workplace engagement. These programs use a bottom-up approach to engage participants as key stakeholders (Mintzberg 1997; Montgomery 2014). Examples include physician well-being committees to launch initiatives, share strategies, and monitor programs longitudinally (Linzer et al. 2009; Linzer et al. 2014; Shannon 2013; Spickard et al. 2002). Positive impacts on burnout last up to one year postintervention. Refresher courses and combined individual-organizational approaches also report favorable sustainable effects on burnout (Awa et al. 2010).

Successful programs demonstrate:

High quality, relevance, and wide applicability
Easy access

Open communication
Strategic alignment with organizational goals
Leadership engagement at every organizational level
Intramural and extramural partnerships to maximize offerings
(Berry, Mirabito, and Baun 2010; Linzer et al. 2009).

National wellness initiatives

Collaborative for Healing and Renewal in Medicine (CHARM) is a collaborative learning community within the Alliance for Academic Internal Medicine (AAIM) to combat issues of burnout in the medical education community. CHARM supports research in learner burnout, assembles tools for medical educators, disseminates best practices, and champions for the acknowledgment and inclusion of well-being initiatives in medical education (AAIM n.d.).

American College of Physicians (ACP) Wellness Champions is a train-the-trainer collaborative addressing physician burnout. Mark Linzer, M.D., a national expert in physician burnout, mentors and trains a cohort of 10 to 12 ACP leaders to educate others on cost-effective strategies and best practices to prevent burnout and foster well-being. The goal is a zero percent rate of burnout among internists and subspecialists ("no physician burnout" motto) and within clinical practices and health care systems. Similar to CHARM, there is no published outcome data for ACP's Wellness Champions (ACP 2017). The Association of Chiefs and Leaders of General Internal Medicine (ACLGIM) created the Wellness Engaged Longitudinal Leaders (WELL) Program to expand the cohort of trained wellness executive champions among primary care and hospitalist physicians (ACLGIM n.d.).

At the advice of her division chief, Deborah met regularly with a psychologist and psychiatrist at her institutional Employee Assistance Program where she learned mindfulness techniques and relaxation exercises to cope with her fears. Narrative medicine and appreciative inquiry strategies helped her "refind" meaning in her career as a physician. After six months, her depression symptoms subsided.

Final Thoughts

Coaching within academic institutions

Professional coaching uses the techniques of positive psychology with four core principles—individual empowerment and self-engagement, strength maximization, meaningful guidance, and subjectivity against self-defeating perceptions (Askin 2008; Gazelle et al. 2015). The focus is on personal and professional growth emphasizing that the individual is in control and empowered while the professional coach is the advocate of change. It is an individual-focused, strength-based, and results-driven process to overcome burnout. Sessions occur weekly or biweekly for six to twelve months (Gazelle et al. 2015).

Several medical schools use this approach in their curriculum (Aboalshamat et al. 2015; Bonrath et al. 2015; Schneider et al. 2014). Massachusetts General Hospital's pioneering program pairs medicine residents with trained faculty coaches to use preassigned session guides (see sample in Appendix) for in-person quarterly meetings that reflect on the residents' performance and growth, capitalizing on strengths and achievements while setting realistic goals for each year (Palamara et al. 2015; Kerri Palamara, personal communication July 22, 2016).

Unfortunately, the evidence on physician coaching is scant. Most studies examined peer-coaching interventions rather than true professional coaching. Modest improvements in communication skills, patient care, practice management, and leadership development were seen (Gattellari et al. 2005; Iyasere et al. 2016; Chase et al. 2015; Egener 2008; Henochowicz and Hetherington 2006; Marr and Kusy 1993). Medical students had short-term reductions in stress and improvements in mental health, but no benefits in academic performance (Aboalshamat et al. 2015; Holm et al. 2010). Among residents, the perception of burnout was lower (Palamara et al. 2015). To date, only one study reported professional coaching decreased burnout among attending physicians (Schneider et al. 2014).

Questions for Future Research

Research designs need longitudinal designs, larger samples, and outcomes of academic and work performance. They should also target interventions at each educational stage of the learner. Other research questions are:

What are the best practices to promote well-being among health professionals?

What specific faculty development programs are the most efficacious?

References

Aach, R., Cooney, T., Girard, D., Grob, D., McCue, J., Page, M., . . . Smith, J. W. (1988). Stress and impairment during residency training: Strategies for reduction, identification, and management. *Annals of Internal Medicine* 109(2): 154–161. doi: 10.7326/0003–4819–109–2-154.

Aboalshamat, K., Hou, X., and Strodl, E. (2015). The impact of a self-development coaching programme on medical and dental students' psychological health and academic performance: A randomised controlled trial. *BMC Medical Education* 15(1). doi: 10.1186/s12909–015–0412–4.

Alliance for Academic Internal Medicine (AAIM). (n.d.). *Collaborative for Healing and Renewal in Medicine (CHARM)*. Retrieved from http://www.im.org/p/cm/ld/fid=1403.

American College of Physicians. (2017). *Physician Burnout and Wellness Information and Resources*. Retrieved from https://www.acponline.org/about-acp/chapters-regions/united-states/new-mexico-chapter/physician-burnout-and-wellness-information-and-resources.

Askin, W. J. (2008). Coaching for physicians: Building more resilient doctors. *Canadian Family Physician* 54(10): 1399–1400.

Association of Chiefs and Leaders of General Internal Medicine (ACLGIM). (n.d.). *ACLGIM WELL Program*. Retrieved from http://www.sgim.org/aclgim-tools—programs/well-program.

Awa, W. L., Plaumann, M., and Walter, U. (2010). Burnout prevention: A review of intervention programs. *Patient Education and Counseling* 78(2): 184–190. doi: 10.1016/j.pec.2009.04.008.

Bar-Sela, G., Lulav-Grinwald, D., and Mitnik, I. (2012). "Balint Group" meetings for oncology residents as a tool to improve therapeutic communication skills and reduce burnout level. *Journal of Cancer Education* 27(4): 786–789. doi: 10.1007/s13187–012–0407–3.

Benbassat, J., Baumal, R., Chan, S., and Nirel, N. (2011). Sources of distress during medical training and clinical practice: Suggestions for reducing their impact. *Medical Teacher* 33(6): 486–490. doi: 10.3109/0142159x.2010.531156.

Berry, L. L., Mirabito, A. M., and Baun, W. B. (2010). What's the hard return on employee wellness programs? *Harvard Business Review* 88(12): 104–12, 142.

Bittner, J. G., 4th, Khan, Z., Babu, M., and Hamed, O. (2011). Stress, burnout, and maladaptive coping: Strategies for surgeon well-being. *Bulletin of the American College of Surgeons* 96(8): 17–22.

Bond, A. R., Mason, H. F., Lemaster, C. M., Shaw, S. E., Mullin, C. S., Holick, E. A., and Saper, R. B. (2013). Embodied health: The effects of a mind-body course for medical students. *Medical Education Online* 18: 1–8. doi: 10.3402/meo.v18i0.20699.

Bonrath, E. M., Dedy, N. J., Gordon, L. E., and Grantcharov, T. P. (2015). Comprehensive surgical coaching enhances surgical skill in the operating room. *Annals of Surgery* 262(2): 205–212. doi: 10.1097/sla.0000000000001214.

Bovier, P. A., and Perneger, T. V. (2007). Stress from uncertainty from graduation to retirement—A population-based study of Swiss physicians. *Journal of General Internal Medicine* 22(5): 632–638. doi: 10.1007/s11606-007-0159-7.

Bushe, G. (1995). Advances in appreciative inquiry as an organizational development intervention. *Organization Development Journal* 13(3): 14–22.

Campbell, J., Prochazka, A. V., Yamashita, T., and Gopal, R. (2010). Predictors of persistent burnout in internal medicine residents: A prospective cohort study. *Academic Medicine* 85(10): 1630–1634. doi: 10.1097/acm.0b013e3181f0c4e7.

Cedfeldt, A. S., Bower, E., Flores, C., Brunett, P., Choi, D., and Girard, D. E. (2015). Promoting resident wellness: Evaluation of a time-off policy to increase residents' utilization of health care services. *Academic Medicine* 90(5): 678–683. doi: 10.1097/acm.0000000000000541.

Centers for Disease Control and Prevention (CDC). (2016). *How is well-being defined?* Retrieved from https://www.cdc.gov/hrqol/wellbeing.htm#three.

Charon, R. (2001). The patient-physician relationship. Narrative medicine: A model for empathy, reflection, profession, and trust. *JAMA* 286(15): 1897. doi: 10.1001/jama.286.15.1897.

Charon, R. (2007). What to do with stories: The sciences of narrative medicine. *Canadian Family Physician* 53(8): 1265–1267.

Chase, S. M., Crabtree, B. F., Stewart, E. E., Nutting, P. A., Miller, W. L., Stange, K. C., and Jaén, C. R. (2015). Coaching strategies for enhancing practice transformation. *Family Practice* 32(1): 75–81. doi: 10.1093/fampra/cmu062.

Collier, V. U., McCue, J. D., Markus, A., and Smith, L. (2002). Stress in medical residency: Status quo after a decade of reform? *Annals of Internal Medicine* 136(5): 384. doi: 10.7326/0003-4819-136-5-200203050-00011.

Conley, C. S., Durlak, J. A., and Kirsch, A. C. (2015). A meta-analysis of universal mental health prevention programs for higher education students. *Prevention Science* 16(4): 487–507. doi: 10.1007/s11121-015-0543-1.

Dabrow, S., Russell, S., Ackley, K., Anderson, E., and Fabri, P. J. (2006). Combating the stress of residency: One school's approach. *Academic Medicine* 81(5): 436–439. doi: 10.1097/01.acm.0000222261.47643.d2.

Daskivich, T. J., Jardine, D. A., Tseng, J., Correa, R., Stagg, B. C., Jacob, K. M., and Harwood, J. L. (2015). Promotion of wellness and mental health awareness among physicians in training: Perspective of a national, multispecialty panel of residents and fellows. *Journal of Graduate Medical Education* 7(1): 143–147. doi: 10.4300/jgme-07-01-42.

de Vibe, M., Solhaug, I., Tyssen, R., Friborg, O., Rosenvinge, J. H., Sørlie, T., and Bjørndal, A. (2013). Mindfulness training for stress management: A randomised controlled study of medical and psychology students. *BMC Medical Education* 13(1). doi: 10.1186/1472-6920-13-107.

Diener, E. (2000). Subjective well-being: The science of happiness and a proposal for a national index. *American Psychologist*, 55(1): 34–43. doi: 10.1037//0003-066x.55.1.34.

Dunn, P. M., Arnetz, B. B., Christensen, J. F., and Homer, L. (2007). Meeting the imperative to improve physician well-being: Assessment of an innovative program. *Journal of General Internal Medicine*, 22(11): 1544–1552. doi: 10.1007/s11606-007-0363-5.

Dyrbye, L., and Shanafelt, T. (2016). A narrative review on burnout experienced by medical students and residents. *Medical Education* 50(1): 132–149. doi: 10.1111/medu.12927.

Eckleberry-Hunt, J., Lick, D., Boura, J., Hunt, R., Balasubramaniam, M., Mulhem, E., and Fisher, C. (2009). An exploratory study of resident burnout and wellness. *Academic Medicine*, 84(2): 269–277. doi: 10.1097/acm.0b013e3181938a45.

Egener, B. (2008). Addressing Physicians' Impaired Communication Skills. *Journal of General Internal Medicine*, 23(11): 1890–1895. doi: 10.1007/s11606-008-0778-7

Eneroth, M., Gustafsson Sendén, M., Løvseth, L. T., Schenck-Gustafsson, K., and Fridner, A. (2014). A comparison of risk and protective factors related to suicide ideation among residents and specialists in academic medicine. *BMC Public Health* 14: 271. doi: 10.1186/1471-2458-14-271

Epstein, R. M., and Krasner, M. S. (2013). Physician resilience: What it means, why it matters, and how to promote it. *Academic Medicine* 88(3): 301–303. doi: 10.1097/acm.0b013e318280cff0.

Erogul, M., Singer, G., Mcintyre, T., and Stefanov, D. G. (2014). Abridged mindfulness intervention to support wellness in first-year medical students. *Teaching and Learning in Medicine* 26(4): 350–356. doi: 10.1080/10401334.2014.945025.

Fares, J., Al Tabosh, H. A., Saadeddin, Z., El Mouhayyar, C. E., and Aridi, H. (2016). Stress, burnout and coping strategies in preclinical medical students. *North American Journal of Medical Sciences* 8(2): 75. doi: 10.4103/1947-2714.177299.

Firth-Cozens, J. (2001). Interventions to improve physicians' well-being and patient care. *Social Science and Medicine* 52(2): 215–222. doi: 10.1016/s0277-9536(00)00221-5.

Ford, C. V., and Wentz, D. K. (1984). The internship year: A study of sleep, mood states, and psychophysiologic parameters. *Southern Medical Journal* 77(11): 1435–1442. doi: 10.1097/00007611-198411000-00019.

Gardiner, P., Filippelli, A. C., Lebensohn, P., and Bonakdar, R. (2015). The incorporation of stress management programming into family medicine residencies—results of a national survey of residency directors: A CERA study. *Family Medicine* 47(4): 272–278.

Gattellari, M., Donnelly, N., Taylor, N., Meerkin, M., Hirst, G., and Ward, J. E. (2005). Does "peer coaching" increase GP capacity to promote informed decision making about PSA screening? A cluster randomised trial. *Family Practice* 22(3): 253–265. doi: 10.1093/fampra/cmi028.

Gazelle, G., Liebschutz, J. M., and Riess, H. (2015). Physician burnout: Coaching a way out. *Journal of General Internal Medicine* 30(4): 508–513. doi: 10.1007/s11606-014-3144-y.

Gerrity, M. S., Devellis, R. F., and Earp, J. A. (1990). Physicians' reactions to uncertainty in patient care: A new measure and new insights. *Medical Care* 28(8): 724–725. doi: 10.1097/00005650-199008000-00005.

Goldman, M. L., Shah, R. N., and Bernstein, C. A. (2015). Depression and suicide among physician trainees: Recommendations for a national response. *JAMA Psychiatry* 72(5): 411–412. doi: 10.1001/jamapsychiatry.2014.3050.

Greenhalgh, T., and Hurwitz, B. (1999). Narrative based medicine: Why study narrative? *BMJ* 318(7175): 48–50. doi: 10.1136/bmj.318.7175.48.

Greeson, J. M., Toohey, M. J., and Pearce, M. J. (2015). An adapted, four-week mind-body skills group for medical students: Reducing stress, increasing mindfulness, and enhancing self-care. *EXPLORE: Journal of Science and Healing* 11(3): 186–192. doi: 10.1016/j.explore.2015.02.003.

Henochowicz, S., and Hetherington, D. (2006). Leadership coaching in health care. *Leadership and Organization Development Journal, 27*(3): 183–189. doi: 10.1108/01437730610657703.

Hirschfeld, R. M., and Klerman, G. L. (1979). Personality attributes and affective disorders. *American Journal of Psychiatry* 136(1): 67–70. doi: 10.1176/ajp.136.1.67.

Hochberg, M. S., Berman, R. S., Kalet, A. L., Zabar, S. R., Gillespie, C., and Pachter, H. L. (2013). The stress of residency: Recognizing the signs of depression and suicide in you and your fellow residents. *American Journal of Surgery* 205(2): 141–146. doi: 10.1016/j.amjsurg.2012.08.003.

Holm, M., Tyssen, R., Stordal, K. I., and Haver, B. (2010). Self-development groups reduce medical school stress: A controlled intervention study. *BMC Medical Education* 10(1). doi: 10.1186/1472-6920-10-23.

Ishak, W. W., Lederer, S., Mandili, C., Nikravesh, R., Seligman, L., Vasa, M., . . . Bernstein, C. A. (2009). Burnout during residency training: A literature review. *Journal of Graduate Medical Education* 1(2): 236–242. doi: 10.4300/jgme-d-09-00054.1.

Iyasere, C. A., Baggett, M., Romano, J., Jena, A., Mills, G., and Hunt, D. P. (2016). Beyond continuing medical education: Clinical coaching as a tool for ongoing professional development. *Academic Medicine* 91(12): 1647–1650. doi: 10.1097/acm.0000000000001131.

Jain, S., Shapiro, S. L., Swanick, S., Roesch, S. C., Mills, P. J., Bell, I., and Schwartz, G. E. (2007). A randomized controlled trial of mindfulness meditation versus relaxation training: Effects on distress, positive states of mind, rumination, and distraction. *Annals of Behavioral Medicine* 33(1): 11–21. doi: 10.1207/s15324796abm3301_2.

Joules, N., Williams, D. M., and Thompson, A. W. (2014). Depression in resident physicians: A systematic review. *Open Journal of Depression* 03(03): 89–100. doi: 10.4236/ojd.2014.33013.

Kalitzkus, V. and Matthiessen, P. F. (2009). Narrative-based medicine: Potential, pitfalls, and practice. *Permanente Journal* 13(1): 80–86. doi: 10.7812/tpp/08–043.

Kemper, K. J., and Yun, J. (2014). Group online mindfulness training proof of concept. *Journal of Evidence-Based Complementary and Alternative Medicine* 20(1): 73–75. doi: 10.1177/2156587214553306.

Kiken, L. G., Garland, E. L., Bluth, K., Palsson O. S., and Gaylord, S. A. (2015, July 1). From a state to a trait: Trajectories of state mindfulness in meditation during intervention predict changes in trait mindfulness. *Personality and Individual Differences* 81: 41–46.

Kimo Takayesu, J., Ramoska, E. A., Clark, T. R., Hansoti, B., Dougherty, J., Freeman, W., . . . Gross, E. (2014). Factors associated with burnout during emergency medicine residency. *Academic Emergency Medicine* 21(9): 1031–1035. doi: 10.1111/acem.12464.

Kraemer, K. M., Luberto, C. M., O'Bryan, E. M., Mysinger, E., and Cotton, S. (2016). Mind-body skills training to improve distress tolerance in medical students: A pilot study. *Teaching and Learning in Medicine* 28(2): 219–228. doi: 10.1080/10401334.2016.1146605.

Krasner, M. S., Epstein, R. M., Beckman, H., Suchman, A. L., Chapman, B., Mooney, C. J., and Quill, T. E. (2009). Association of an educational program in mindful communication with burnout, empathy, and attitudes among primary care physicians. *JAMA* 302(12): 1284. doi: 10.1001/jama.2009.1384.

Lemkau, J. P., Purdy, R. R., Rafferty, J. P., and Rudisill, J. R. (1988). Correlates of burnout among family practice residents. *Journal of Medical Education* 63(9): 682–691. doi: 10.1097/00001888–198809000–00003.

Levin, S., Aronsky, D., Hemphill, R., Han, J., Slagle, J., and France, D. J. (2007). Shifting toward balance: Measuring the distribution of workload among emergency physician teams. *Annals of Emergency Medicine* 50(4): 419–423. doi: 10.1016/j.annemergmed.2007.04.007.

Linzer, M., Levine, R., Meltzer, D., Poplau, S., Warde, C., and West, C. P. (2014). 10 bold steps to prevent burnout in general internal medicine. *Journal of General Internal Medicine* 29(1): 18–20. doi: 10.1007/s11606–013–2597–8.

Linzer, M., Manwell, L. B., Williams, E. S., Bobula, J. A., Brown, R. L., Varkey, A. B., . . . MEMO (Minimizing Error, Maximizing Outcome) Investigators (2009). Working conditions in primary care: Physician reactions and care quality. *Annals of Internal Medicine* 151(1): 28–36. doi: 10.7326/0003–4819–151–1–200907070–00006.

Longenecker, R., Zink, T., and Florence, J. (2012). Teaching and learning resilience: Building adaptive capacity for rural practice. A report and subsequent analysis of a workshop conducted at the Rural Medical Educators Conference, Savannah, Georgia, May 18, 2010. *Journal of Rural Health* 28(2): 122–127. doi: 10.1111/j.1748–0361.2011.00376.x.

Maclaughlin, B. W., Wang, D., Noone, A., Liu, N., Harazduk, N., Lumpkin, M., . . . Amri, H. (2011). Stress biomarkers in medical students participating in a mind body medicine skills program. *Evidence-Based Complementary and Alternative Medicine* 2011: 1–8. doi: 10.1093/ecam/neq039.

Marr, T. J., and Kusy, M. E., Jr. (1993). Building physician managers and leaders: A model. *Physician Executive* 19(2): 30–32.

Martini, S., Arfken, C. L., Churchill, A., and Balon, R. (2004). Burnout comparison among residents in different medical specialties. *Academic Psychiatry* 28(3): 240–242. doi: 10.1176/appi.ap.28.3.240.

Maslach, C., Jackson, S. E., and Leiter, M. P. (1996). *Maslach burnout inventory manual* (3rd ed.). Palo Alto, CA: Consulting Psychologists Press.

McCranie, E. W., and Brandsma, J. M. (1989). Personality antecedents of burnout among middle-aged physicians. *Hospital Topics* 67(4): 32–37. doi: 10.1080/00185868 .1989.10543667.

McCray, L. W., Cronholm, P. F., Bogner, H. R., Gallo, J. J., and Neill, R. A. (2008). Resident physician burnout: Is there hope? *Family Medicine* 40(9): 626–632.

McNeeley, M. F., Perez, F. A., and Chew, F. S. (2013). The emotional wellness of radiology trainees: Prevalence and predictors of burnout. *Academic Radiology* 20(5): 647–655. doi: 10.1016/j.acra.2012.12.018.

Mintzberg, H. (1997). Toward healthier hospitals. *Health Care Management Review* 22(4): 9–18. doi: 10.1097/00004010-199710000-00005.

Montgomery, A. (2014). The inevitability of physician burnout: Implications for interventions. *Burnout Research* 1(1): 50–56. doi: 10.1016/j.burn.2014.04.002.

Morris, D. B. (1993). *The culture of pain*. Oakland, CA: University of California Press.

Moutier, C., Norcross, W., Jong, P., Norman, M., Kirby, B., Mcguire, T., and Zisook, S. (2012). The Suicide Prevention and Depression Awareness Program at the University of California, San Diego School of Medicine. *Academic Medicine* 87(3): 320–326. doi: 10.1097/acm.0b013e31824451ad.

Nes, R. B., Røysamb, E., Tambs, K., Harris, J. R., and Reichborn-Kjennerud, T. (2006). Subjective well-being: Genetic and environmental contributions to stability and change. *Psychological Medicine* 36(7): 1033–1042. doi: 10.1017/s0033291706007409.

Novack, D. H., Epstein, R. M., and Paulsen, R. H. (1999). Toward creating physician-healers: Fostering medical students' self-awareness, personal growth, and well-being. *Academic Medicine* 74(5): 516–520. doi: 10.1097/00001888-199905000-00017.

Novack, D. H., Suchman, A. L., Clark, W., Epstein, R. M., Najberg, E., and Kaplan, C. (1997). Calibrating the physician. Personal awareness and effective patient care. Working Group on Promoting Physician Personal Awareness, American Academy on Physician and Patient. *JAMA: Journal of the American Medical Association* 278(6): 502–509. doi: 10.1001/jama.278.6.502.

Palamara, K., Kauffman, C., Stone, V. E., Bazari, H., and Donelan, K. (2015). Promoting success: A professional development coaching program for interns in medicine. *Journal of Graduate Medical Education* 7(4): 630–637. doi: 10.4300/jgme-d-14-00791.1.

Paulson, S., Davidson, R., Jha, A., and Kabat-Zinn, J. (2013). Becoming conscious: The science of mindfulness. *Annals of the New York Academy of Sciences* 1303(1): 87–104. doi: 10.1111/nyas.12203.

Pololi, L., and Frankel, R. M. (2001). Small-group teaching emphasizing reflection can positively influence medical students' values. *Academic Medicine* 76(12): 1172; author reply 1172–1173. doi: 10.1097/00001888-200112000-00002.

Prins, J. T., Gazendam-Donofrio, S. M., Tubben, B. J., van der Heijden, F. M., van de Wiel, H. B., and Hoekstra-Weebers, J. E. (2007). Burnout in medical residents: A review. *Medical Education* 41(8): 788–800. doi: 10.1111/j.1365-2923.2007.02797.x.

Purdy, R. R., Lemkau, J. P., Rafferty, J. P., and Rudisill, J. R. (1987). Resident physicians in family practice: Who's burned out and who knows? *Family Medicine* 19(3): 203–208.

Ramanan, R. A., Taylor, W. C., Davis, R. B., and Phillips, R. S. (2006). Mentoring matters. Mentoring and career preparation in internal medicine residency training. *Journal of General Internal Medicine* 21(4): 340–345. doi: 10.1111/j.1525–1497.2006.00346.x.

Reynolds, C. F., 3rd, and Clayton, P. J. (2009). Commentary: Out of the silence: Confronting depression in medical students and residents. *Academic Medicine* 84(2): 159–160. doi: 10.1097/acm.0b013e31819397c7.

Ripp, J., Babyatsky, M., Fallar, R., Bazari, H., Bellini, L., Kapadia, C., . . . Korenstein, D. (2011). The incidence and predictors of job burnout in first-year internal medicine residents: A five-institution study. *Academic Medicine* 86(10): 1304–1310. doi: 10.1097/acm.0b013e31822c1236.

Romani, M., and Ashkar, K. (2014). Burnout among physicians. *Libyan Journal of Medicine* 9(1): 23556. doi: 10.3402/ljm.v9.23556.

Rosenzweig, S., Reibel, D. K., Greeson, J. M., Brainard, G. C., and Hojat, M. (2003). Mindfulness-based stress reduction lowers psychological distress in medical students. *Teaching and Learning in Medicine* 15(2): 88–92. doi: 10.1207/s15328015tlm1502_03.

Rutherford, K., and Oda, J. (2014). Family medicine residency training and burnout: A qualitative study. *Canadian Medical Education Journal* 5(1): e13–23.

Sargent, M. C., Sotile, W., Sotile, M. O., Rubash, H., and Barrack, R. L. (2004). Stress and coping among orthopaedic surgery residents and faculty. *Journal of Bone and Joint Surgery-American* 86(7): 1579–1586. doi: 10.2106/00004623–200407000–00032.

Satterfield, J. M., and Becerra, C. (2010). Developmental challenges, stressors and coping strategies in medical residents: A qualitative analysis of support groups. *Medical Education* 44(9): 908–916. doi: 10.1111/j.1365–2923.2010.03736.x.

Schneider, S., Kingsolver, K., and Rosdahl, J. (2014). Physician coaching to enhance well-being: A qualitative analysis of a pilot intervention. *EXPLORE: Journal of Science and Healing* 10(6): 372–379. doi: 10.1016/j.explore.2014.08.007

Schrijver, I. (2016). Pathology in the Medical Profession?: Taking the Pulse of Physician Wellness and Burnout. *Archives of Pathology and Laboratory Medicine, 140*(9): 976–982. doi: 10.5858/arpa.2015–0524-ra.

Schultz, J. H., and Luthe, W. (1959). *Autogenic training: A psychophysiologic approach in psychotherapy*. New York, NY: Grune & Stratton.

Seligman, M. E., Steen, T. A., Park, N., and Peterson, C. (2005). Positive psychology progress: Empirical validation of interventions. *American Psychologist* 60(5): 410–421. doi: 10.1037/0003–066x.60.5.410.

Shanafelt, T. D. (2009). Enhancing meaning in work: A prescription for preventing physician burnout and promoting patient-centered care. *JAMA* 302(12): 1338–1340. doi: 10.1001/jama.2009.1385.

Shanafelt, T. D., Bradley, K. A., Wipf, J. E., and Back, A. L. (2002). Burnout and self-reported patient care in an internal medicine residency program. *Annals of Internal Medicine* 136(5): 358. doi: 10.7326/0003–4819–136–5–200203050–00008.

Shannon, D. (2013). Physician well-being: A powerful way to improve the patient experience. *Physician Executive* 39(4): 6–8, 10, 12.

Shapiro, S. L., Shapiro, D. E., and Schwartz, G. E. (2000). Stress management in medical education: A review of the literature. *Academic Medicine* 75(7): 748–759. doi: 10.1097/00001888-200007000-00023.

Sheikhmoonesi, F., and Zarghami, M. (2014). Prevention of physicians' suicide. *Iranian Journal of Psychiatry and Behavioral Sciences* 8(2): 1–3.

Sheldon, K. M., and Lyubomirsky, S. (2006). How to increase and sustain positive emotion: The effects of expressing gratitude and visualizing best possible selves. *Journal of Positive Psychology* 1(2): 73–82. doi: 10.1080/17439760500510676.

Spickard, J. A., Jr., Gabbe, S. G., and Christensen, J. F. (2002). Mid-career burnout in generalist and specialist physicians. *JAMA* 288(12): 1447–1450. doi: 10.1001/jama .288.12.1447.

Thomas, N. K. (2004). Resident burnout. *JAMA* 292(23): 2880. doi: 10.1001/jama.292.23 .2880.

Veldenz, H. C., Scott, K. K., Dennis, J. W., Tepas, J. J., and Schinco, M. S. (2003). Impaired residents: Identification and intervention. *Current Surgery* 60(2): 214–217. doi: 10.1016/s0149-7944(02)00780-8.

Wald, H. S. (2015). Professional identity (trans)formation in medical education: Reflection, relationship, resilience. *Academic Medicine* 90(6): 701–706. doi: 10.1097/ acm.0000000000000731.

Wallace, J. E., Lemaire, J. B., and Ghali, W. A. (2009). Physician wellness: A missing quality indicator. *Lancet* 374(9702): 1714–1721. doi: 10.1016/s0140-6736(09)61424-0.

West, C. P., Dyrbye, L. N., Rabatin, J. T., Call, T. G., Davidson, J. H., Multari, A., ... Shanafelt, T. D. (2014). Intervention to Promote Physician Well-being, Job Satisfaction, and Professionalism. *JAMA Internal Medicine, 174*(4): 527–533. doi: 10.1001/ jamainternmed.2013.14387

Wild, K., Scholz, M., Ropohl, A., Bräuer, L., Paulsen, F., and Burger, P. H. (2014). Strategies against burnout and anxiety in medical education—Implementation and evaluation of a new course on relaxation techniques (Relacs) for medical students. *PLoS ONE* 9(12). doi: 10.1371/journal.pone.0114967.

Winkel, A. F., Hermann, N., Graham, M. J., and Ratan, R. B. (2010). No time to think: Making room for reflection in obstetrics and gynecology residency. *Journal of Graduate Medical Education* 2(4): 610–615. doi: 10.4300/jgme-d-10-00019.1.

Zwack, J., and Schweitzer, J. (2013). If every fifth physician is affected by burnout, what about the other four? Resilience strategies of experienced physicians. *Academic Medicine* 88(3): 382–389. doi: 10.1097/acm.0b013e318281696b.

Additional Resources

Finding Meaning in Medicine: http://www.ishiprograms.org/programs/all-healthcare-professionals/

Civility, Respect and Engagement at Work: http://www.workengagement.com/

Mindfulness in Medicine: http://www.fammed.wisc.edu/mindfulness/

2

Medical Error and Resilience

MARYAM SATTARI, JAMES SMITH, AND ROBERT WATSON[1]

Errare humanum est—To err is human, or, everybody makes mistakes.
Seneca

In this chapter, we discuss the intersection of medical errors and medical fallibility and their relationship to burnout and resilience using a clinical vignette of a preventable medical error. In addition, we review curricula on improving resilience.

Objectives

Recognize the systemic and personal impact of medical errors.
Define medical fallibility and its relationship to medical errors.
Define resilience and burnout.
Discuss curricula for improving resilience as it relates to medical errors.

A 46-year-old man presents to the emergency department (ED) with severe headache and weakness. He has fever, photophobia, neck stiffness, and generalized weakness. Laboratory studies reveal leukopenia, anemia, hypokalemia, hypoalbuminemia, and increased gamma globulin antibody fraction. After neuroimaging and lumbar puncture, the ED physician starts treatment for "classic cryptococcal meningitis" and admits the patient to the teaching medicine team. Later that day, staff find the patient unre-

1 Maryam Sattari, M.D., M.S., University of Florida College of Medicine, Gainesville, FL.
James Smith, M.D., University of Florida College of Medicine, Gainesville, FL.
Robert Watson, M.D., Florida State University College of Medicine, Tallahassee, FL.

sponsive and in ventricular fibrillation. He does not survive despite the team's resuscitation attempts.

The attending physician discusses the case with team members individually and informs them that the hypokalemia was a contributing factor to the ventricular fibrillation. The medical student tells the attending that a repeat potassium level was pending. The intern discloses that she attributed the presenting symptoms to the meningitis, missed the hypokalemia on admission, and had not ordered potassium replacement or a repeat level. The senior resident confides that he only learned of the hypokalemia while reviewing the labs in the team room. He had called the ED nurse and verbally ordered potassium repletion with a repeat level, but forgot to enter the orders into the electronic medical record.

The Toll of Medical Errors

Medical errors affect 50 percent of hospitalized patients and are responsible for considerable morbidity, mortality, and health care costs (T. A. Brennan et al. 1991; Zhan and Miller, 2003; Rothschild et al. 2005; Baker et al. 2004). In the United States, preventable medical errors contribute to 40,000–90,000 deaths annually (Kohn et al. 1999; Singh et al. 2012). In addition, one in 20 primary care visits involves a preventable diagnostic error, half of which are potentially harmful (Kohn et al. 1999; Singh et al. 2012). In other words, preventable medical errors harm an average of 10 patients in our clinics or emergency rooms every day, resulting in an average of 10 deaths per hospital annually.

What Is Medical Fallibility?

Medical fallibility is the *unintentional* likelihood of making errors (Vincent et al. 1989). Nonmedical professions, such as the airline industry, confirm some degree of error is inherent in all human activity (Perrow 1984), and medicine is no exception (Kohn et al. 1999; Vincent et al. 2001; AAMC: Joint Committee 2003; Volpp and Grande 2003; Schenkel et al. 2003). It is distinct from negligence, which "occurs not merely when there is error, but when the degree of error exceeds an accepted norm. The presence of error is a necessary but insufficient condition for the determination of negligence" (Leape et al. 1991, p. 381).

Etiologies of Medical Errors

Sleepiness, fatigue, depression, stress, burnout, reduced quality of life, communication errors, and handoff problems increase the risk of future self-perceived and self-reported medical errors (Jagsi et al. 2005; Kohn et al. 1999; Landrigan et al. 2004; Barger et al. 2006; Lockley et al. 2007; West et al. 2006; Fahrenkopf et al. 2008; Lockley et al. 2004). The association between resident work hours and medical fallibility is inconsistent (Bilimoria et al. 2016; Philibert et al. 2013). Other contributing factors include suboptimal coordination of multiple caregivers, inadequate resident supervision, dependence on diagnoses made by inexperienced clinicians, inadequate input by consultants, and lack of detailed patient assessments prior to discharge (Neale et al. 2001). Interestingly, physicians' self-perceived error rates do not vary significantly by their age, sex, relationship status, program type, amount of student loan debt, or parental status (West et al. 2009). While surgical trainees are more likely to report adverse events (AEs) than medical trainees, the proportion of AEs attributed to errors do not vary significantly by specialty (Jagsi et al. 2005).

Diagnostic errors (missed, delayed, or wrong diagnosis) are either no fault, system-related, or cognitive (Graber et al. 2005). System-related factors include policy- or procedure-related problems; inadequate supervision; and inefficient processes, teamwork, and communication. Cognitive problems include inadequate knowledge, faulty synthesis, premature closure (failure to consider reasonable alternatives after the initial diagnosis), faulty context generation, misjudgment of salient findings, faulty perception, and heuristical errors (Graber et al. 2005).

Prevention of Medical Errors

The Institute of Medicine recommends a systems-level approach focused on effective teamwork for reducing medical errors (National Academies of Sciences, Engineering, and Medicine 2015). They also advocate for curricula and training at each career stage to address performance in the diagnostic process, including the incorporation of clinical reasoning, teamwork communication, diagnostic testing, and health information technology. The health professional's ability to generate an appropriate differential diagnosis is the cornerstone for reducing errors (Bordage 1999; Singh et al. 2013). Trowbridge et al. (2013) propose that practicing health professionals and learners focus on metacognition, intuitive reasoning, and the recognition of the role of systems in diagnostic errors. Other important skills are communicating effectively, reflecting, recognizing when to slow down and ask for help, and working effectively in interdisciplinary teams (Trowbridge et al. 2013).

Responding to Medical Errors

Disclosing unanticipated outcomes to patients is a core component of high-quality health care, and health professionals must possess the knowledge and skills to successfully execute this task (Gallagher et al. 2007). Ideally, error disclosure includes a frank conversation using plain language, provides details regarding the error, discusses any future necessary medical care, and includes an "expression of regret for unanticipated outcomes" with a straightforward and honest apology for the error (Gallagher et al. 2013; Gallagher et al. 2007). Reviewing the error, identifying its cause(s), and solving any systems-related issues reduce the risk of future harm. Furthermore, health professionals should report medical errors in a timely manner to their institution's quality assurance department, risk management group, and/or malpractice carrier.

Culture Is the Key

Only 10 percent of physicians surveyed agreed that health care organizations supported them in coping with medical errors (Waterman et al. 2007). Fear of punishment limits early event reporting to institutions and disclosure to patients and families. Creating and sustaining a rigorous sense of professional accountability without adding blame or shame to the emotional burdens of learners and physicians involved in medical errors foster a safety culture and encourage open reporting of error (Gallagher et al. 2007). Organizational resources can support physicians' and learners' self-identities as healers while they navigate the psychological demands of the disclosure process and its aftermath. Furthermore, organizational support encourages physicians to communicate with patients and families about errors, promotes the dignity and well-being of the harmed patient, and enhances transparency in health care (Kohn et al. 1999; Leape et al. 2002).

Teaching about Medical Fallibility

Medical educators are responsible for preparing learners to prevent and recognize medical errors, report and disclose errors, address and minimize the negative consequences of errors, and perform systems-based root-cause analysis. Trowbridge (2008) proposes a framework for familiarizing learners with the common causes of diagnostic errors, and simple strategies to avoid errors. Strategies include recognizing heuristics and their impact on clinical reasoning, performing diagnostic time-outs, practicing worst-case-scenario medicine, using a systematic approach to common problems, embracing "zebras" (rare or exotic medical diagnoses in medicine), asking why, valuing the clinical exam, using Bayesian theory, acknowledging how the patient makes the clinician feel, slowing down, and admitting one's own mistakes (Trowbridge 2008).

The emotional impact of medical errors differentiates them from other clinical experiences (M. A. Fischer et al. 2006). Formal, longitudinal, evidence-based curricula addressing medical errors and disclosure should begin early in the medical curriculum. Major themes include learning from errors and near misses; the emotional and cognitive impact of errors and apologies on patients, physicians, and teams; effective and ineffective apologies; and the balance between individual and systems responsibility. Integrating actual error cases and faculty disclosure into curricula addresses both learner knowledge and the hidden curriculum. Involving learners in quality improvement (QI) initiatives, patient-safety programs, and root-cause analysis encourages them to identify errors in their own work and enhances their professional development (Sorokin et al. 2005; Volpp and Grande 2003; Van Eaton et al. 2005).

Existing Curricula

Currently, only a few medical schools provide formal instruction in error and disclosure (Hafferty 1998; S. M. Fischer et al. 2003; Wong et al. 2010), which may lead to physicians entering practice unprepared for the challenges of disclosure and unable to accept their own fallibility.

1. Learners

Most learners report personal involvement with errors (Gallagher et al. 2006; Mizrahi 1984), but felt ill-prepared (White et al. 2008). Most formal curricula involve either medical students or residents from a single institution, and used multiple teaching modalities (Table 2). The curricula were well accepted, and learners demonstrated improved knowledge and attitudes toward medical errors (Wong et al. 2010) and safety-related behaviors (Ahmed et al. 2014). Learners noted discrepancies between curricular material and their local institutional practice or culture (Wong et al. 2010). Successful programs addressed competing educational demands, ensured learners' buy-in and enthusiasm, and included adequate faculty familiar with QI and patient safety content (Wong et al. 2010).

2. Faculty

Faculty may lack training on how to respond to learners' errors, highlighting the need for faculty development curricula in medical errors (Mazor et al. 2005). Preceptors who teach from their own experiences or "wing it" might not be comfortable giving corrections, or may avoid explicit feedback when discussing errors (Ende et al. 1995; Burack et al. 1999). Faculty training in errors and disclosure facilitates effective mentoring of trainees (Shojania et al. 2006), and should include training in how to provide effective, explicit, and corrective feedback in response to learners' errors and near misses, as well as how to identify AEs due to negligence. In addition, it is crucial to recognize that guilt, self-doubt, isolation, and vulnerability after an error are very real for learners, even in the absence of external criticism. Frank discussions with supervising faculty can reduce inappropriate self-blame and distress and prevent future errors (West et al. 2009; Waterman et al. 2007). Faculty should encourage learners to accept responsibility, discuss their mistakes, and seek support when worried about errors. In addition, sharing personal experience about medical errors promotes learning while providing mentorship. Faculty role modeling of error disclosure accelerates learners' recognition that errors accompany even the best clinical efforts, while emphasizing that error disclosure is a normal component of respectful patient care.

Table 2. Modalities and topics of formal medical fallibility and error disclosure curricula

Modalities

Anonymous feedback by peers on written apologies (Gillies et al. 2011)

Case investigation/root-cause analysis (Thompson et al. 2008; Coyle 2005; Gunderson et al. 2009; Ahmed et al. 2014)

Case/team-based discussion/learning (Varkey 2007; Newell et al. 2008; Ahmed et al. 2014)

Conference (Coyle 2005; Ahmed et al. 2014)

Lecture (Fischer et al. 2006; Varkey 2007; Thompson et al. 2008; Coyle 2005; Gunderson et al. 2009; Halbach and Sullivan 2005a; Patey et al. 2007; Gillies et al. 2011)

Exercise-based discussions (Varkey 2007)

Experiential learning (Thompson et al. 2008; Ahmed et al. 2014)

Facilitated discussion (Gunderson et al. 2009)

Grand rounds (Fischer et al. 2006)

Interactive didactic (Gunderson et al. 2009)

Interdisciplinary rounds/shadowing (Thompson et al. 2008)

Learning exercises (Gillies et al. 2011)

Modeling/observation (Gillies et al. 2011; Thompson et al. 2008)

Morbidity and mortality conferences (Fischer et al. 2006; Orlander et al. 2002; Pierluissi et al. 2003)

Orientation activities (Fischer et al. 2006)

OSCE (Fischer et al. 2006; Varkey 2007)

Panel discussions (Meyer 1989)

Patient safety course/elective (Varkey 2007; Thompson et al. 2008; Gunderson et al. 2009)

Plenary sessions (Gunderson et al. 2009; Moskowitz et al. 2007)

Practicing responding to and discussing errors and apologies with peers, superiors, or patients (Gillies et al. 2011)

Readings (Halbach and Sullivan, 2005b; Gunderson et al. 2009; Newell et al. 2008; Meyer 1989)

Reflection/debriefing sessions (Gunderson et al. 2009; Halbach and Sullivan, 2005b)

Role play (Thompson et al. 2008; Gunderson et al. 2009; Patey et al. 2007; Moskowitz et al. 2007)

Courses (entire course or integrated into a course) (Fischer et al. 2006; Gillies et al. 2011; Thompson et al. 2008)

Seminar (Thompson et al. 2008)

Simulations (Varkey 2007)

Small and large group case discussions (Fischer et al. 2006; Halbach and Sullivan 2005b; Coyle 2005; Gunderson et al. 2009; Patey et al. 2007; Meyer 1989; Newell et al. 2008; Gillies et al. 2011; Ahmed et al. 2014)

Standardized patients (Halbach and Sullivan 2005b; Varkey 2007; Gunderson et al. 2009; Gillies et al. 2011)

Student presentations (Thompson et al. 2008; Ahmed et al. 2014)

Team projects (Thompson et al. 2008)

Video (Varkey, 2007; Thompson et al. 2008; Halbach and Sullivan, 2005b; Patey et al. 2007; Coyle, 2005; Gunderson et al. 2009; Patey et al. 2007; Gillies et al. 2011)

Web-based modules (Gillies et al. 2011; Patey et al. 2007)

Workshops (Moskowitz et al. 2007)

Topics/Objectives Reported in the Curricula

AES

Factors influencing AEs (Ahmed et al. 2014)

Investigating an AE (Thompson et al. 2008)

APOLOGIZING

Impact of apologies (Gillies et al. 2011)

Suggestions for effective apologies (Gillies et al. 2011; Thompson et al. 2008; Gunderson et al. 2009)

The 4 "Rs" of apology: recognition, responsibility, regret, and remedy (Gunderson et al. 2009)

Clinical QI (Thompson et al. 2008; Gunderson et al. 2009; Moskowitz et al. 2007)

Evidence-based practice (Thompson et al. 2008)

INTERDISCIPLINARY TEAM COLLABORATION

Definition of team (Moorman 2005)

Effective communication (Varkey 2007; Thompson et al. 2008; Gunderson et al. 2009; Patey et al. 2007; Moskowitz et al. 2007; Moorman 2005)

Teamwork/effective collaboration (Varkey 2007; Thompson et al. 2008; Moorman 2005)

Techniques of conflict resolution (Moorman 2005)

MEDICAL ERRORS

Active vs. latent errors (Patey et al. 2007)

Causes/factors contributing to errors (Coyle 2005; Ahmed et al. 2014; Patey et al. 2007; Moskowitz et al. 2007)

Cognitive error (Ahmed et al. 2014)

Coping/dealing with error (Patey et al. 2007; Gillies et al. 2011)

Definition of errors (Patey et al. 2007)

Disclosure (Varkey 2007; Thompson et al. 2008; Patey et al. 2007; Madigosky et al. 2006; Moskowitz et al. 2007; Coyle 2005; Gunderson et al. 2009)

Impact of errors (Patey et al. 2007; Coyle 2005; Gillies et al. 2011; Ahmed et al. 2014; Moskowitz et al. 2007; Moorman 2005)

Models/classification of error (Patey et al. 2007)

Prevention of errors (Coyle, 2005; Patey et al. 2007; Ahmed et al. 2014; Moskowitz et al. 2007; Moorman 2005)

Rates of errors/patient safety incidents (Ahmed et al. 2014; Patey et al. 2007)

Reflecting and learning from errors (Ahmed et al. 2014; Patey et al. 2007)

(continued)

Table 2—*Continued*

Reporting errors (Thompson et al. 2008; Coyle 2005; Patey et al. 2007; Moskowitz et al. 2007)

Types of errors (Newell et al. 2008; Patey et al. 2007)

Near misses (Coyle 2005)

PATIENT SAFETY

Identification of hazards in patient care that pose risks to patient safety (Thompson et al. 2008)

Impact of culture, including teamwork and communication, on patient safety (Thompson et al. 2008; Patey et al. 2007)

Institute of Medicine quality aims/core competencies (Thompson et al. 2008)

Legal aspects of patient safety (Patey et al. 2007; Moskowitz et al. 2007)

Patient-centered care (Thompson et al. 2008)

Patient safety improvement tools (Thompson et al. 2008)

Patient safety overview (Thompson et al. 2008; Gillies et al. 2011)

Patient safety skills and attitudes (Ahmed et al. 2014)

Root-cause analysis (Varkey 2007; Thompson et al. 2008; Coyle,, 2005; Gunderson et al. 2009; Ahmed et al. 2014; Moorman 2005)

SAFETY CULTURE

Avoiding blame/shame (Gillies et al. 2011)

Focusing on cause rather than culprit (Patey et al. 2007)

Fostering an open and learning culture to improve patient safety (Ahmed et al. 2014)

Improving teamwork and assertive communication (Thompson et al. 2008)

Supporting others involved in errors (Patey et al. 2007)

SYSTEMS

Systems-based defects (Thompson et al. 2008)

Systems' impact on patient safety and quality (Ahmed et al. 2014; Patey et al. 2007)

Systems theory (Moskowitz et al. 2007; Thompson et al. 2008)

System vs. human approach (Thompson et al. 2008; Patey et al. 2007; Ahmed et al. 2014)

Compiled by authors.
Abbreviations
AE = Adverse event
OSCE = Simulation/objective structured clinical examination
QI = Quality improvement

Case Discussion

The case of ventricular fibrillation in the setting of untreated hypokalemia represents a preventable medical error. The attending physician used this error to discuss cognitive and system-based contributors to the error, patient safety, and error disclosure (Figure 2). Each learner acknowledges an error has occurred, accepts responsibility, and discusses the error and

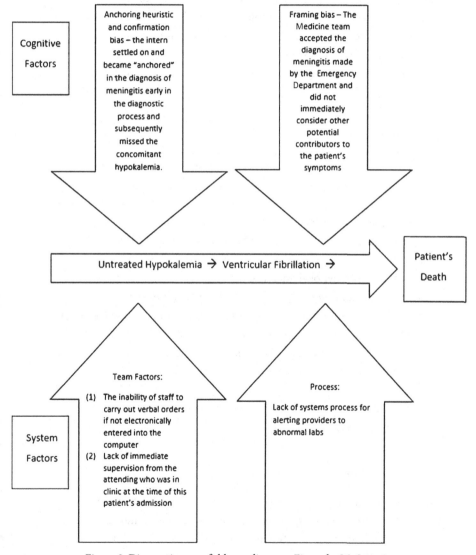

Figure 2. Diagnostic error fishbone diagram. Figure by M. Sattari.

its impact. The attending physician should review with the student and intern the importance of reporting the accurate status of a laboratory test, as well as the clinical manifestations and consequences of hypokalemia. With the resident, the attending physician may discuss causes of the error, future error prevention, and error disclosure to the patient's family, while role-modeling error disclosure to the patient's family for the entire team. This example reinforces that a physician's obligation is to inform patients of all aspects of their medical care, even when mistakes occur. Sharing individual experiences of preventable errors and disclosures that went well or poorly further reinforces the culture of transparency in medicine. Also, the attending physician should inform the institution's quality assurance department, risk management group, and/or malpractice carrier of the error.

Case Continued

A few months later, the ED attending physician reports several hostile interactions with the intern. Other residents note she is defensive and "hyper-conscientious"—the first to come in and the last to leave, double-checking labs and orders to make sure she does not miss anything. Others report she is sarcastic, cynical, "less fun to be around," and does not socialize with them. The tipping point in the intern's behavior was the loss of her patient with hypokalemia. The resident involved in the case has also changed. He continues to socialize after-hours and exercise, but he now routinely discusses recognition and management of common electrolyte abnormalities with his entire team the first day of each rotation. Additionally, he became involved in a QI project with the aim of improving communication and handoffs between the ED and Medicine service.

Both the intern and the resident were involved in the same case. Is the resident more resilient?

What Is Resilience?

Resilience is the "ability to adapt in the face of tragedy, trauma, adversity, hardship, and ongoing significant life stressors" (Newman 2005, p. 227). Siebert's Resiliency Model (Siebert 2005) describes five key behaviors of a resilient individual:

Managing health
Problem solving
Increasing self-strengths including self-esteem, self-confidence, and
    self-concept
Developing positive response choices
Learning good lessons from demanding situations

Medical training is a time of significant growth and adaptation, as well as stress. There is a daunting amount of material to learn, and professional identities to develop. There is the stress of preparing for licensure, and the added challenge of interacting with patients, families, and other health care team members. Learners progress to their residency training, where they face increased patient care responsibility and autonomy. Significant conflicts can develop in balancing professional and personal lives. After residency, as practicing physicians, they face the challenges of bearing the ultimate responsibility for their patients, as well as competing demands for their professional and personal time. Each of these transitions poses increased stress for the learner.

What Is Burnout?

Burnout is a state of emotional exhaustion, a low sense of personal accomplishment and associated diminished effectiveness at work, and depersonalization (Shanafelt et al. 2002). Burnout relates to a person's work, while depression affects a person's life more globally (Shanafelt et al. 2002). Fifteen to 20 percent of physicians experience mental health problems during their careers (Boisaubin and Levine 2001). Cohen et al. (2008) found that one third of residents reported their life was "quite a bit" or "extremely" stressful. Kjeldstadli et al. (2006) found that life satisfaction among entering medical students was not different from age-matched university student controls; however, it was significantly less in their final year of training. Dyrbye et al. (2006) found 45 percent of medical students in Minnesota met criteria for burnout based on the Maslach Burnout Inventory (Maslach et al. 1986). The increase in sense of personal accomplishment produced by years of training was offset by an increase in depersonalization; 35 percent exhibited high emotional exhaustion. They also found a high rate of depressive symptoms (56 percent) and at-risk alcohol use (22 percent) (Dyrbye et al. 2006).

How Do Resilience and Burnout Relate to Medical Errors?

There is limited evidence about the relationship of resilience, burnout, and depression with medical errors. Fahrenkopf et al. (2008) found depressed residents made more medical errors than nondepressed residents; however, there was no association between burnout and medical errors. The Iatroref study involving ICU staff reported similar findings (Garrouste-Orgeas et al. 2015). In contrast, others found an association between burnout and medical errors (Prins et al. 2009; Kang et al. 2013). Perceived medical errors were more common in residents who screened positive for depression and among those with higher levels of fatigue and distress (West et al. 2009). Thus, efforts to improve learners' quality of life and reduce burnout may have a positive effect on medical errors.

Resilience fluctuates based on the situation. Individuals can learn and enhance their resilience. In contrast, hardiness is a stable personality trait (Egeland et al. 1993). Dunn et al. (2008) propose a conceptual model of well-being, where medical students' personality and temperament ("hardiness") influence their coping reserve. Negative and positive inputs further affect their coping reserve. Negative inputs include stress, internal conflict, and time and energy demands. Positive inputs include psychosocial support, social activities, mentorship, and intellectual stimulation. Through the interactions of baseline characteristics and the balance of positive and negative inputs, learners develop either burnout or well-being (Dunn et al. 2008). (Refer to Chapter 1, "Focusing on Well-Being," for a complete review of strategies to promote well-being and resilience.)

Existing Curricula

1. Learners

Thomas et al. (2011) implemented and evaluated a didactic curriculum covering mental health, help seeking, and stress resilience to volunteer first-year medical students. Student feedback indicated that the presentations were interesting and provided information useful to maintaining balance during medical school. Responses varied as to whether each presentation provided information relevant to future practice. The study did not assess resiliency.

Hassed et al. (2009) studied the effects of a Health Enhancement Program on first-year medical students using a curriculum of eight lectures followed by six two-hour small group tutorials. The program showed improvements in the depression and hostility components of the Symptom Checklist-90-R and in the WHO Quality of Life questionnaire. A daily 30-minute audio mindfulness practice for eight weeks led to improved Perceived Stress Scale scores and ratings on the anxiety component of the Depression, Anxiety, and Stress Scale (Warnecke et al. 2011).

Brennan and McGrady (2015) reported on a resiliency program for family medicine residents that incorporated interactive sessions covering multiple topics including: introduction to wellness and resiliency, the importance of spending time with family and balancing work and home life, positive psychology, mindfulness, time management/stress coping, and outdoor team building. They found moderate levels of burnout in their residents based on the Maslach Burnout Inventory. Residents found the sessions to be useful, and increased their frequency of exercise and healthier diets.

Another study utilizing two to three hours of mindfulness-based activities did not show a significant difference in the Depression Anxiety Stress Scale (DASS-21) scores, although there was a trend toward reduced scores in females and in the postgraduate years one and two (Goldhagen et al. 2015). In a study of burnout in critical care fellows, Kashani et al. (2015) found no significant improvements in burnout after a single, 90-minute intervention; however, the fellows felt that they had learned tools that were useful in stressful situations.

2. Faculty

A 90-minute group session utilizing the Stress Management and Resiliency Training (SMART) program with two follow-up phone interviews resulted in significant improvements in perceived stress, anxiety, quality of life, and mindfulness among radiology faculty after 12 weeks (Sood et al. 2014). However, there were no differences in resilience scores between the intervention and control groups. Kemper and Khirallah (2015) reported significant improvement in stress reduction, mindfulness, resilience, and empathy after a one-hour online mind-body skills training program. West et al. (2014) conducted an intensive intervention involving

19 biweekly discussion groups over a nine-month period. Discussion topics included mindfulness, reflection, shared experience, and small group learning. They noted increases in empowerment and engagement at work as well as decreased rates of depersonalization, emotional exhaustion, and overall burnout; improvements were sustained at 12 months.

Krasner et al. (2009) studied 70 primary care physicians who underwent an intensive 52-hour intervention and saw improvements in mindfulness, burnout, empathy, physician belief scale, personality, and total mood disturbance. Similarly, after eight weeks of 60–90-minute interventions, Internal Medicine faculty showed significant improvements in resilience, anxiety, and overall quality of life (Sood et al. 2011).

Case Discussion

The loss of their patient deeply affected and changed the intern and the resident in the clinical case. However, the same stressors that led to burnout in one did not in the other. The resident's resilience and his efforts to prevent future errors are laudable. For the intern, the residency program should take the opportunity to recognize her burnout and offer support. In addition to screening for depression and anxiety, and counseling to help her deal with the loss of her patient, she would benefit from interventions to enhance her resilience. The program should facilitate her access to medical appointments by allowing her time off during clinical hours, and also encourage her to get adequate rest; engage in extracurricular activities; and cultivate relationships with colleagues, family, and friends. Early intervention will increase her self-esteem, self-confidence, and self-concept, while helping her acquire the skills to manage her own health, problem-solve, develop positive response choices, and learn "good lessons from difficult situations." These skills will foster her well-being and resilience during training and over the course of her career.

Final Thoughts

Medical errors are inevitable events that offer educators important teachable moments about both patient safety and disclosing errors to patients (Hilfiker 1984; Mazor et al. 2005; Leape 2005; Leape 2006; Berlinger 2003). Although medical errors are only one of the factors that contribute to the stressful milieu for learners in medical education, they lead to a high rate of burnout, depression, and substance abuse in trainees and practicing physicians. Currently, only a limited number of interventions have successfully enhanced resilience and wellness.

Questions for Future Research

Do interventions that result in sustainable reductions in medical errors, stress, and/or burnout also improve patient outcomes and physician well-being and/or resilience?

What is the ideal model for framing educational efforts to improve resiliency as it relates to medical errors?

When is the optimal time to introduce resiliency programs in medical education?

How should we address volunteer bias and choose appropriate controls?

References

Ahmed, M., Arora, S., Tiew, S., Hayden, J., Sevdalis, N., Vincent, C., and Baker, P. (2014). Building a safer foundation: The Lessons Learnt patient safety training programme. *BMJ Quality and Safety* 23(1), 78–86. doi: 10.1136/bmjqs-2012–001740.

Association of American Medical Colleges (AAMC): Joint Committee of the Group on Resident Affairs and Organization of Resident Representatives. (2003). Patient Safety and Graduate Medical Education. Retrieved July 14, 2017, from https://members.aamc.org/eweb/upload/patient%20safety%20gme.pdf.

Baker, G. R., Norton, P.G., Flintoff, V., Blais, R., Brown, A., Cox, J., . . . Tamblyn, R. (2004). The Canadian Adverse Events Study: The incidence of adverse events among hospital patients in Canada. *Canadian Medical Association Journal* 170(11): 1678–1686. doi: 10.1503/cmaj.1040498.

Barger, L. K., Ayas, N. T., Cade, B. E., Cronin, J. W., Rosner, B., Speizer, F. E., and Czeisler, C. A. (2006). Impact of extended-duration shifts on medical errors, adverse events, and attentional failures. *PLoS Medicine,* 3(12): e487. doi: 10.1371/journal.pmed.0030487.

Berlinger, N. (2003). Avoiding cheap grace: Medical harm, patient safety, and the culture(s) of forgiveness. *Hastings Center Report* 33(6): 28–36. doi: 10.2307/3527823.

Bilimoria, K. Y., Chung, J. W., Hedges, L. V., Dahlke, A. R., Love, R., Cohen, M. E., . . . Lewis, F. R. (2016). National cluster-randomized trial of duty-hour flexibility in surgical training. *New England Journal of Medicine* 374(8): 713–727. doi: 10.1056/nejmoa1515724.

Boisaubin, E. V., and Levine, R. E. (2001). Identifying and assisting the impaired physician. *American Journal of the Medical Sciences* 322(1): 31–36. doi: 10.1097/00000441-200107000-00006.

Bordage, G. (1999). Why did I miss the diagnosis? Some cognitive explanations and educational implications. *Academic Medicine* 74(10): S138–43. doi: 10.1097/00001888-199910000-00065.

Brennan, T. A. Leape, L. L., Laird, N. M., Herbert, L., Localio, A. R., Lawthers, A. G., . . . Hiatt, H. H. (1991). Incidence of adverse events and negligence in hospitalized patients: Results of the Harvard Medical Practice Study I. *New England Journal of Medicine* 324(6): 370–376. doi: 10.1056/NEJM199102073240604.

Brennan, J., and McGrady, A. (2015). Designing and implementing a resiliency program for family medicine residents. *International Journal of Psychiatry in Medicine* 50(1): 104–114. doi: 10.1177/0091217415592369.

Burack, J. H., Irby, D. M., Carline, J. D., Root, R. K., and Larson, E. B. (1999). Teaching compassion and respect: Attending physicians' responses to problematic behaviors. *Journal of General Internal Medicine* 14(1): 49–55. doi: 10.1046/j.1525-1497.1999.00280.x.

Cohen, J. S., Leung, Y., Fahey, M., Hoyt, L., Sinha, R., Cailler, L., . . . Patten, S. (2008). The happy docs study: A Canadian Association of Internes and Residents well-being survey examining resident physician health and satisfaction within and outside of residency training in Canada. *BMC Research Notes* 1(1): 105. doi: 10.1186/1756-0500-1-105.

Coyle, Y. M. (2005). Effectiveness of a graduate medical education program for improving medical event reporting attitude and behavior. *Quality and Safety in Health Care* 14(5): 383–388. doi: 10.1136/qshc.2005.013979.

Dunn, L. B., Iglewicz, A., and Moutier, C. (2008). A conceptual model of medical student well-being: Promoting resilience and preventing burnout. *Academic Psychiatry* 32(1): 44–53. doi: 10.1176/appi.ap.32.1.44.

Dyrbye, L. N., Thomas, M. R., Huntington, J. L., Lawson, K. L., Novotny, P. J., Sloan, J. A., and Shanafelt, T. D. (2006). Personal life events and medical student burnout: A multicenter study. *Academic Medicine* 81(4): 374–384. doi: 10.1097/00001888-200604000-00010.

Egeland, B., Carlson, E., and Sroufe, L. A. (1993). Resilience as process. *Development and Psychopathology* 5(04): 517–528. doi: 10.1017/s0954579400006131.

Ende, J., Pomerantz, A., and Erickson, F. (1995). Preceptors' strategies for correcting residents in an ambulatory care medicine setting. *Academic Medicine* 70(3): 224–229. doi: 10.1097/00001888-199503000-00014.

Fahrenkopf, A. M., Sectish, T. C., Barger, L. K., Sharek, P. J., Lewin, D., Chiang, V. W., . . . Landrigan, C. P. (2008). Rates of medication errors among depressed and burnt out residents: Prospective cohort study. *BMJ* 336(7642): 488–491. doi: 10.1136/bmj.39469.763218.be.

Fischer, M. A., Mazor, K. M., Baril, J., Alper, E., DeMarco, D., and Pugnaire, M. (2006). Learning from mistakes: Factors that influence how students and residents learn from medical errors. *Journal of General Internal Medicine* 21(5): 419–423. doi: 10.1111/j.1525–1497.2006.00420.x.

Fischer, S. M., Gozansky, W. S., Kutner, J. S., Chomiak, A., and Kramer, A. (2003). Palliative care education: An intervention to improve medical residents' knowledge and attitudes. *Journal of Palliative Medicine* 6(3): 391–399.

Gallagher, T. H., Denham, C., Leape, L., Amori, G., and Levinson, W. (2007). Disclosing unanticipated outcomes to patients: The art and the practice. *Journal of Patient Safety* 3, 158–165.

Gallagher, T. H., Garbutt, J. M., Waterman, A. D., Flum, D. R., Larson, E. B., Waterman, B. M., . . . Levinson, W. (2006). Choosing your words carefully: How physicians would disclose harmful medical errors to patients. *Archives of Internal Medicine* 166(15): 1585–1593. doi: 10.1001/archinte.166.15.1585.

Gallagher, T. H., Mello, M. M., Levinson, W., Wynia, M. K., Sachdeva, A. K., Sulmasy, L. S., . . . Arnold, R. (2013). Talking with patients about other clinicians' errors. *New England Journal of Medicine* 369(18): 1752–1757. doi: 10.1056/nejmsb1303119.

Gallagher, T. H., Studdert, D., and Levinson, W. (2007). Disclosing harmful medical errors to patients. *New England Journal of Medicine* 356(26): 2713–2719. doi: 10.1056/nejmra070568.

Gallagher, T. H., Waterman, A. D., Garbutt, J. M., Kapp, J. M., Chan, D. K., Dunagan, W. C., . . . Levinson, W. (2006). US and Canadian physicians' attitudes and experiences regarding disclosing errors to patients. *Archives of Internal Medicine* 166(15): 1605–1611. doi: 10.1001/archinte.166.15.1605.

Garrouste-Orgeas, M., Perrin, M., Soufir, L., Vesin, A., Blot, F., Maxime, V., . . . Timsit, J. (2015). The Iatroref study: Medical errors are associated with symptoms of depression in ICU staff but not burnout or safety culture. *Intensive Care Medicine* 41(2): 273–284. doi: 10.1007/s00134-014-3601-4.

Gillies, R. A., Speers, S., Young, S. E., and Fly, C. A. (2011). Teaching medical error apologies: Development of a multi-component intervention. *Family Medicine* 43(6): 400–406.

Goldhagen, B. E., Kingsolver, K., Stinnett, S. S., and Rosdahl, J. A. (2015). Stress and burnout in residents: Impact of mindfulness-based resilience training. *Advances in Medical Education and Practice* (6): 525–532. doi: 10.2147/AMEP.S88580.

Graber, M. L., Franklin, N., and Gordon, R. (2005). Diagnostic error in internal medicine. *Archives of Internal Medicine* 165(13): 1493–1499. doi: 10.1001/archinte.165.13.1493.

Gunderson, A. J., Smith, K. M., Mayer, D. B., McDonald, T., and Centomani, N. (2009). Teaching medical students the art of medical error full disclosure: Evaluation of a new curriculum. *Teaching and Learning in Medicine* 21(3): 229–232. doi: 10.1080/10401330903018526.

Hafferty, F. W. (1998). Beyond curriculum reform: Confronting medicine's hidden curriculum. *Academic Medicine* 73(4): 403–407. doi: 10.1097/00001888-199804000-00013.

Halbach, J., and Sullivan, L. (2005a). Medical errors and patient safety: A curriculum guide for teaching medical students and family practice residents. *MedEdPORTAL Publications* (1): 101. doi: 10.15766/mep_2374-8265.101.

Halbach, J. L., and Sullivan, L. L. (2005b). Teaching medical students about medical errors and patient safety: Evaluation of a required curriculum. *Academic Medicine* 80(6): 600–606. doi: 10.1097/00001888-200506000-00016.

Hassed, C., de Lisle, S., Sullivan, G., and Pier, C. (2009). Enhancing the health of medical students: Outcomes of an integrated mindfulness and lifestyle program. *Advances in Health Sciences Education* 14(3): 387–398. doi: 10.1007/s10459-008-9125-3.

Hevia, A., and Hobgood, C. (2003). Medical error during residency: To tell or not to tell. *Annals of Emergency Medicine* 42(4): 565–570. doi: 10.1067/s0196-0644(03)00399-8.

Hilfiker, D. (1984). Facing our mistakes. *New England Journal of Medicine* 310(2): 118–122. doi: 10.1056/nejm198401123100211.

Jagsi, R., Kitch, B. T., Weinstein, D. F., Campbell, E. G., Hutter, M., and Weissman, J. S. (2005). Residents report on adverse events and their causes. *Archives of Internal Medicine* 165(22): 2607–2613. doi: 10.1001/archinte.165.22.2607.

Kang, E., Lihm, H., and Kong, E. (2013). Association of intern and resident burnout with self-reported medical errors. *Korean Journal of Family Medicine* 34(1): 36–42. doi: 10.4082/kjfm.2013.34.1.36.

Kashani, K., Carrera, P., Moraes, A. G., Sood, A., Onigkeit, J. A., and Ramar, K. (2015). Stress and burnout among critical care fellows: Preliminary evaluation of an educational intervention. *Medical Education Online* 20(1): 27840. doi: 10.3402/meo.v20.27840.

Kemper, K. J., and Khirallah, M. (2015). Acute effects of online mind-body skills training on resilience, mindfulness, and empathy. *Journal of Evidence-Based Complementary and Alternative Medicine* 20(4): 247–253. doi: 10.1177/2156587215575816.

Kjeldstadli, K., Tyssen, R., Finset, A., Hem, E., Gude, T., Gronvold, N. T., . . . Vaglum, P. (2006). Life satisfaction and resilience in medical school—A six-year longitudinal, nationwide and comparative study. *BMC Medical Education* 6(1). doi: 10.1186/1472-6920-6-48.

Kohn, L. T., Corrigan, J., and Donaldson, M. S. (eds.). (1999). *To err is human: Building a safer health system.* Washington, D.C.: National Academy Press.

Krasner, M. S., Epstein, R. M., Beckman, H., Suchman, A. L., Chapman, B., Mooney, C. J., and Quill, T. E. (2009). Association of an educational program in mindful communication with burnout, empathy, and attitudes among primary care physicians. *JAMA* 302(12): 1284–1293. doi: 10.1001/jama.2009.1384.

Landrigan, C. P., Rothschild, J. M., Cronin, J. W., Kaushal, R., Burdick, E., Katz, J. T., . . . Czeisler, C. A. (2004). Effect of reducing interns' work hours on serious medical errors in intensive care units. *New England Journal of Medicine* 351(18): 1838–1848.

Leape, L. L. (2005). Understanding the power of apology: How saying "I'm sorry" helps heal patients and caregivers. *Focus on Patient Safety* 8(4): 1–3.

Leape, L. L. (2006). Full disclosure and apology—an idea whose time has come. *Physician Executive* 32(2): 16–18.

Leape, L. L., Berwick, D. M., and Bates, D. W. (2002). What practices will most improve safety? *JAMA* 288(4): 501–507. doi: 10.1001/jama.288.4.501.

Leape, L. L., Brennan, T. A., Laird, N., Lawthers, A. G., Localio, A. R., Barnes, B. A., . . . Hiatt, H. (1991). The nature of adverse events in hospitalized patients. Results of the

Harvard Medical Practice Study II. *New England Journal of Medicine* 324(6): 377–384. doi: 10.1056/NEJM199102073240605.

Lockley, S. W., Barger, L. K., Ayas, N. T., Rothschild, J. M., Czeisler, C. A., Landrigan, C. P., Harvard Work Hours, Health and Safety Group. (2007). Effects of health care provider work hours and sleep deprivation on safety and performance. Joint Commission *Journal on Quality and Patient Safety* 33(Suppl. 11): 7–18.

Lockley, S. W., Cronin, J. W., Evans, E. E., Cade, B. E., Lee, C. J., Landrigan, C. P., . . . Harvard Work Hours, Health and Safety Group. (2004). Effect of reducing interns' weekly work hours on sleep and attentional failures. *New England Journal of Medicine* 351(18): 1829–1837. doi: 10.1056/NEJMoa041404.

Madigosky, W. S., Headrick, L. A., Nelson, K., Cox, K. R., and Anderson, T. (2006). Changing and sustaining medical students' knowledge, skills, and attitudes about patient safety and medical fallibility. *Academic Medicine* 81(1): 94–101. doi: 10.1097/00001888-200601000-00022.

Maslach, C., Jackson, S. E., and Leiter, M. P. (1986). Maslach Burnout Inventory. Palo Alto, CA: Consulting Psychologists Press.

Mazor, K. M., Fischer, M. A., Haley, H., Hatem, D., and Quirk, M. E. (2005). Teaching and medical errors: Primary care preceptors' views. *Medical Education* 39(10): 982–990. doi: 10.1111/j.1365-2929.2005.02262.x.

Meyer, B. A. (1989). A student teaching module: Physician errors. *Family Medicine* 21(4): 299–300.

Mizrahi, T. (1984). Managing medical mistakes: Ideology, insularity and accountability among internists-in-training. *Social Science and Medicine* 19(2): 135–146. doi: 10.1016/0277-9536(84)90280-6.

Moorman, D. W. (2005). On the quest for Six Sigma. *American Journal of Surgery* 189(3): 253–258. doi: 10.1016/j.amjsurg.2004.11.027.

Moskowitz, E., Veloski, J. J., Fields, S. K., and Nash, D. B. (2007). Development and evaluation of a 1-day interclerkship program for medical students on medical errors and patient safety. *American Journal of Medical Quality* 22(1): 13–17. doi: 10.1177/1062860606296669.

National Academies of Sciences, Engineering, and Medicine. (2015). Improving diagnosis in health care. Washington, DC: National Academies Press. https://doi.org/10.17226/21794.

Neale, G., Woloshynowych, M., and Vincent, C. (2001). Exploring the causes of adverse events in NHS hospital practice. *Journal of the Royal Society of Medicine* 94(7): 322–330.

Newell, P., Harris, S., Aufses, A., and Ellozy, S. (2008). Student perceptions of medical errors: Incorporating an explicit professionalism curriculum in the third-year surgery clerkship. *Journal of Surgical Education* 65(2): 117–119. doi: 10.1016/j.jsurg.2008.02.005.

Newman, R. (2005). APA's Resilience Initiative. *Professional Psychology: Research and Practice* 36(3): 227–229. doi: 10.1037/0735-7028.36.3.227.

Orlander, J. D., Barber, T. W., and Fincke, B. G. (2002). The Morbidity and Mortality Conference. *Academic Medicine* 77(10): 1001–1006. doi: 10.1097/00001888-200210000-00011.

Patey, R., Flin, R., Cuthbertson, B. H., Macdonald, L., Mearns, K., Cleland, J., and Williams, D. (2007). Patient safety: Helping medical students understand error in healthcare. *Quality and Safety in Health Care* 16(4): 256–259. doi: 10.1136/qshc.2006.021014.

Perrow, C. (1984). Normal accidents: Living with high-risk technologies. New York: Basic Books.

Philibert, I., Nasca, T., Brigham, T., and Shapiro, J. (2013). Duty-hour limits and patient care and resident outcomes: Can high-quality studies offer insight into complex relationships? *Annual Review of Medicine* 64(1): 467–483. doi: 10.1146/annurev-med-120711-135717.

Pierluissi, E., Fischer, M. A., Campbell, A. R., Landefeld, C. S. (2003). Discussion of Medical Errors in Morbidity and Mortality conferences. *JAMA* 290(21): 2838–2342. doi: 10.1001/jama.290.21.2838.

Prins, J. T., van der Heijden, F. M., Hoekstra-Weebers, J. E., Bakker, A. B., van de Wiel, H. B., Jacobs, B., and Gazendam-Donofrio, S. M. (2009). Burnout, engagement and resident physicians' self-reported errors. *Psychology, Health and Medicine* 14(6): 654–666. doi: 10.1080/13548500903311554.

Rothschild, J. M., Landrigan, C. P., Cronin, J. W., Kaushal, R., Lockley, S. W., Burdick, E., . . . Bates, D. W. (2005). The Critical Care Safety Study: The incidence and nature of adverse events and serious medical errors in intensive care. *Critical Care Medicine* 33(8): 1694–1700. doi: 10.1097/01.ccm.0000171609.91035.bd.

Schenkel, S. M., Khare, R., Rosenthal, M., Sutcliffe, K., and Lewton, E. (2003). Resident perceptions of medical errors in the emergency department. *Academic Emergency Medicine* 10(12): 1318–1324. doi: 10.1197/s1069-6563(03)00559-1.

Shanafelt, T. D., Bradley, K. A., Wipf, J. E., and Back, A. L. (2002). Burnout and self-reported patient care in an internal medicine residency program. *Annals of Internal Medicine* 136(5): 358–367. doi: 10.7326/0003-4819-136-5-200203050-00008.

Shojania, K. G., Fletcher, K. E., and Saint, S. (2006). Graduate medical education and patient safety: A busy—and occasionally hazardous—intersection. *Annals of Internal Medicine* 145(8): 592. doi: 10.7326/0003-4819-145-8-200610170-00008.

Siebert, A. (2005). *Resiliency advantage: Master change, thrive under pressure, and bounce back from setbacks.* Readhowyouwant.com.

Singh, H., Giardina, T. D., Forjuoh, S. N., Reis, M. D., Kosmach, S., Khan, M. M., and Thomas, E. J. (2012). Electronic health record-based surveillance of diagnostic errors in primary care. *BMJ Quality and Safety* 21(2): 93–100. doi: 10.1136/bmjqs-2011-000304.

Singh, H., Giardina, T. D., Meyer, A. N., Forjuoh, S. N., Reis, M. D., and Thomas, E. J. (2013). Types and origins of diagnostic errors in primary care settings. *JAMA Internal Medicine* 173(6): 418–425. doi: 10.1001/jamainternmed.2013.2777.

Sood, A., Prasad, K., Schroeder, D., and Varkey, P. (2011). Stress management and resilience training among department of medicine faculty: A pilot randomized clinical trial. *Journal of General Internal Medicine* 26(8): 858–861. doi: 10.1007/s11606-011-1640-x.

Sood, A., Sharma, V., Schroeder, D. R., and Gorman, B. (2014). Stress Management and Resiliency Training (SMART) Program among department of radiology faculty: A pilot randomized clinical trial. *EXPLORE: Journal of Science and Healing* 10(6): 358–363. doi: 10.1016/j.explore.2014.08.002.

Sorokin, R., Riggio, J. M., and Hwang, C. (2005). Attitudes about patient safety: A survey of physicians-in-training. *American Journal of Medical Quality* 20(2): 70–77. doi: 10.1177/1062860604274383.

Thomas, S. E., Haney, M. K., Pelic, C. M., Shaw, D., and Wong, J. G. (2011). Developing a program to promote stress resilience and self-care in first-year medical students. *Canadian Medical Education Journal* 2(1): e32–e36.

Thompson, D. A., Cowan, J., Holzmueller, C., Wu, A. W., Bass, E., and Pronovost, P. (2008). Planning and implementing a systems-based patient safety curriculum in medical education. *American Journal of Medical Quality* 23(4): 271–278. doi: 10.1177/1062860608317763.

Trowbridge, R. L. (2008) Twelve tips for teaching avoidance of diagnostic errors. *Medical Teacher* 30(5):496–500.

Trowbridge, R. L., Dhaliwal, G., and Cosby, K. S. (2013). Educational agenda for diagnostic error reduction. *BMJ Quality & Safety* 22(Suppl. 2): ii28–ii32. doi: 10.1136/bmjqs-2012-001622.

Van Eaton, E. G., Horvath, K. D., Pellegrini, C. A. (2005). Professionalism and the shift mentality: How to reconcile patient ownership with limited work hours. *Archives of Surgery* 140(3): 230–235. doi: 10.1001/archsurg.140.3.230.

Varkey, P. (2007). Educating to improve patient care: Integrating quality improvement into a medical school curriculum. *American Journal of Medical Quality* 22(2): 112–116. doi: 10.1177/1062860606298338.

Vincent, C., Neale, G., and Woloshynowych, M. (2001). Adverse events in British hospitals: Preliminary retrospective record review. *BMJ* 322(7285): 517–519. doi: 10.1136/bmj.322.7285.517.

Vincent, C. A. (1989). Research into medical accidents: A case of negligence? *BMJ* 299(6708): 1150–1153. doi: 10.1136/bmj.299.6708.1150.

Volpp, K. G., and Grande, D. (2003). Residents' suggestions for reducing errors in teaching hospitals. *New England Journal of Medicine* 348(9): 851–855. doi: 10.1056/nejmsb021667.

Warnecke, E., Quinn, S., Ogden, K., Towle, N., and Nelson, M. R. (2011). A randomised controlled trial of the effects of mindfulness practice on medical student stress levels. *Medical Education* 45(4): 381–388. doi: 10.1111/j.1365-2923.2010.03877.x.

Waterman, A. D., Garbutt, J., Hazel, E., Dunagan, W. C., Levinson, W., Fraser, V. J., and Gallagher, T. H. (2007). The emotional impact of medical errors on practicing physicians in the United States and Canada. *Joint Commission Journal on Quality and Patient Safety* 33(8): 467–476. doi: 10.1016/s1553-7250(07)33050-x.

West, C. P., Dyrbye, L. N., Rabatin, J. T., Call, T. G., Davidson, J. H., Multari, A., . . . Shanafelt, T. D. (2014). Intervention to promote physician well-being, job satisfaction, and professionalism: A randomized clinical trial. *JAMA Internal Medicine* 174(4): 527–533. doi: 10.1001/jamainternmed.2013.14387.

West, C. P., Huschka, M. M., Novotny, P. J., Sloan, J. A., Kolars, J. C., Habermann, T. M., and Shanafelt, T. D. (2006). Association of perceived medical errors with resident distress and empathy: A prospective longitudinal study. *JAMA* 296(9): 1071–1078. doi: 10.1001/jama.296.9.1071.

West, C. P., Tan, A. D., Habermann, T. M., Sloan, J. A., and Shanafelt, T. D. (2009). Association of resident fatigue and distress with perceived medical errors. *JAMA* 302(12): 1294–1300. doi: 10.1001/jama.2009.1389.

White, A. A., Gallagher, T. H., Krauss, M. J., Garbutt, J., Waterman, A. D., Dunagan, W. C., . . . Larson, E. B. (2008). The attitudes and experiences of trainees regarding disclosing medical errors to patients. *Academic Medicine* 83(3): 250–256. doi: 10.1097/acm.0b013e3181636e96.

Wong, B. M., Etchells, E. E., Kuper, A., Levinson, W., and Shojania, K. G. (2010). Teaching quality improvement and patient safety to trainees: A systematic review. *Academic Medicine* 85(9): 1425–1439. doi: 10.1097/acm.0b013e3181e2d0c6.

Zhan, C., and Miller, M. R. (2003). Excess length of stay, charges, and mortality attributable to medical injuries during hospitalization. *JAMA* 290(14): 1868–1874. doi: 10.1001/jama.290.14.1868.

3

Attitude and Work Ethic

HENRIQUE KALLAS AND REBECCA J. BEYTH[1]

Labor omnia vincit—Work overcomes all.
Virgil

We developed a conceptual framework using complexity theory to promote a good attitude and work ethic within the health care system and medical education. In addition, we explore the humanistic role of the health professional, and challenges to maintaining a good attitude and work ethic.

Objectives

Describe the intrinsic connection of attitude and work ethic to the humanistic role of a health professional.

Discuss challenges to a good attitude and work ethic.

Provide a framework for understanding how to promote a good attitude and work ethic in medical education.

Recommend tools to aid in promoting a good attitude and work ethic.

Wilbur arrives 30 minutes late for his scheduled appointment at his primary care physician's office. He is 80 years old and lives alone. He has severe visual impairment and quit driving last year. A few weeks ago, he arranged for his neighbor to drive him to this office visit; he has no other means of transportation. He brings all his medicine bottles in a brown bag for his physician, Eleanor, to review. His neighbor has helped him make a list of medical concerns he also wants to discuss. At check-in, the clerk

---

1 Henrique Kallas, M.D., University of Florida College of Medicine, Gainesville, FL.
   Rebecca J. Beyth, M.D., M.Sc. University of Florida College of Medicine, Malcom Randall VA Medical Center, Gainesville, FL.

informs Wilbur of the clinic's policy to reschedule patients who show up more than 20 minutes late. Wilbur is disappointed and frustrated. The clerk notifies Eleanor, who knows of Wilbur's difficulties and suggests she will accommodate him between patients or at the end of clinic if he can wait. She acknowledges his frustration and expresses her appreciation of how difficult it is for him to arrange travel. Wilbur's frustration and disappointment have abated. He thanks Eleanor and the clerk for taking the time and the special attention to his individual needs.

Medicine, along with the law and clergy, is one of the three original learned professions (Freidson 1988). Crucial characteristics of a profession include a specialized body of knowledge and skills, autonomy and self-regulation of the discipline, and a commitment to the public good (Hilton and Southgate 2007). Thus, *expertise, ethics,* and *service* emerged as the three pillars of medical professionalism (Irvine 1997). The roots of professionalism in Western medicine trace back to the times of Apollo and Hippocrates (Porter 1997), with increasing emphasis on developing professionalism as a core goal of medical education. Swick posited that medical professionalism "must be grounded in what physicians actually do and how they act, individually and collectively" (Swick 2000, p. 614).

Inherent in the concept of medical professionalism is the idea that there are virtues that encompass more than technical and knowledge-based competencies. Thus, physicians have the two intertwined roles of healer and professional (R. L. Cruess and Cruess 1997; S. R. Cruess and Cruess 1997; Sohl and Bassford 1986). When one of these roles takes priority over the other, a tension can arise that affects attitude and work ethic. For example, tension may occur when a physician self-recognizes only as a healer and neglects professional duties, such as billing and coding or appropriately managing time. It can also arise from prioritizing only the professional aspects of medicine where the focus is solely on the number of patients seen in a day or increasing a clinic's efficiency. Historically, the balance of healer versus professional has shifted in the eyes of the profession, as well as the public (R. L. Cruess and Cruess 1997). This shift led to a sense of public distrust and a call to return to the "virtues" of the medical profession as a counterbalance to the increasing corporatization of medical practice (Abelson et al. 1997; Blumenthal 1994; Colgan 2014; Haug 1972; Mechanic 1985; Swick 2000). Medical societies have convened to examine and redefine medical professionalism to steer the profession back on course (ABIM Foundation et al. 2002).

The case of Eleanor illustrates a scenario where the physician achieves a balance between her roles as a healer and a professional. As a professional, she is cognizant of her duty to the other patients who are waiting, her office staff, and her practice colleagues. She is also able to exhibit compassion and empathy to Wilbur, whose blindness and dependence on others affected his ability to make his appointment on time. She has consciously chosen to prioritize altruism over self-interest. Hilton and Southgate (2007) note that altruism is the "moral and ethical practice that puts the interest of the client above their own" (p. 267), and the benefit of this altruism is autonomy and self-regulation. Several researchers argue that the changes in both the practice of medicine and the health care industry have led to a loss of autonomy, respect, and morale; health professionals need to renew their social and moral contract with those they serve (R. L. Cruess and Cruess 1997; R. L. Cruess et al. 1999; S. R. Cruess and Cruess 1997; Swick et al. 1999). In contrast, others suggest that the focus should shift to the health care system itself—that is, the context in which health professionals practice (Frankford et al. 2000; Ginsburg et al. 2000; Rothman 2000). Hilton and Southgate (2007) explicitly link this shift toward the context in which health professionals practice to the promotion of "mindful practice" (Epstein 1999) as a strategy to deal with the "technical rationality" of modern medicine that is insufficient for both health professional and the patient.

Humanistic Virtues: The Basis for Good Attitude and Work Ethic

"Honesty, integrity, caring and compassion, altruism and empathy, respect for others, and trustworthiness" are the core humanistic virtues of the medical profession (Swick 2000). As medical educators, we strive to train technically competent health professionals who possess these core humanistic virtues. Patients expect and deserve physicians with an excellent working knowledge of medical science coupled with strong humanistic characteristics and capacities. Arnold and Stern, in *Measuring Medical Professionalism* (2006), describe humanism as one of four pillars of medical professionalism, along with altruism, excellence, and accountability. J. J. Cohen (2007) similarly describes the intimate association between humanism and professionalism: "Humanism provides the passion that animates authentic professionalism. . . . It comprises a set of deep-seated personal convictions about one's obligations to others, especially others in need. Humanistic physicians are intuitively and strongly motivated to adhere to the traditional virtues and expectations of their calling (Cohen 2007, p. 1029). Cohen continues: "Professionalism and humanism are best considered not as separate attributes of a good doctor, but rather as being intimately linked" (Cohen 2007, p. 1031). Thus, despite the many definitions of professionalism (Birden et al. 2014), good attitude and work ethic remain an integral part of the fabric of being a physician along with medical knowledge and clinical competence (Olthuis and Dekkers 2003; Woloschuk et al. 2004). Otherwise, we risk transmitting to our learners "an unreflective mechanical view of professionalism" (Brody and Doukas 2014, p. 981).

In the broadest definition, attitudes are, as Richardson notes, "a predisposition to feel, think, and act towards some object, person, group or event in a more or less favourable or unfavourable way" (as cited in Kelly et al. 2002 p. 206). In medicine, attitude refers more specifically to the "capacity of persons to respond to others in a particular situation in a humane manner" (Olthuis and Dekkers 2003, p. 930). Therefore, attitude connotes a moral component of the way physicians act (Olthuis and Dekkers 2003). Woloschuk et al. (2004) expand the work of Newble (1992) to posit, "Attitude is the mediating link between clinical competence (knowledge and skills) and clinical performance" (Woloschuk et al. 2004 p. 522). Work ethic is another construct linked to attitude and considered a fundamental component of professionalism. Although there is no consensus on the definition of "work ethic," M. J. Miller et al. (2001) note that it is a multidimensional construct reflecting "a constellation of attitudes and beliefs pertaining to work behavior" that is learned, secular, and not specific to any one profession. The existing measures to capture the true essence of what "work ethic" is are incomplete, complicating research efforts in this area (M. J. Miller et al. 2001, p. 5). Work ethic is a "motivational construct reflected in behavior" (M. J. Miller et al. 2001, p. 5), and attitudes influence behavior (Woloschuk et al. 2004). Thus, work ethic and attitude are components of the fabric of what it means to be a physician.

The hidden curriculum of medical education affects the formation of good attitude and professionalism. The hidden curriculum constitutes a set of influences, either positive or negative, at the level of the structure and culture of the institution by which learners acquire the "culture" of their profession (Hafferty and Franks 1994). The detrimental effects of the hidden curriculum profoundly affect medical education (Hafferty and Franks 1994). Anecdotes can perpetuate and reinforce gender, racial, ethnic, and other stereotypes (Hafferty and Franks 1994). Furthermore, these negative influences often represent a significant barrier to effective role modeling (S. R. Cruess et al. 2008). Detrimental effects include the promotion of a culture that deprioritizes collegial interpersonal interactions, empathetic medical care, and quality teaching. Thus, learners may adopt attitudes and work ethics that are the antithesis to the healer role of a physician via enculturation ("the hidden curriculum") and by direct observations of faculty behavior (Hafferty and Franks 1994; Woloschuk et al. 2004).

Challenges to a Good Attitude and Work Ethic

The movement in medicine to a "patient-centered care" approach, where physicians exhibit more humanistic qualities, supports a more balanced approach to the role of a physician as healer and professional (Gerteis et al. 1993; Mead and Bower 2000). Inclusive in the patient-centered approach is "shared decision-making" (Charles et al. 1997), a collaborative process allowing patients and physicians to make health care decisions jointly by reconciling the patient's values and preferences with the best available scientific evidence.

Despite the recognition and growing trend for patient-centered care and shared decision making, other forces in the health care arena challenge the humanistic component of practicing modern medicine. Staying true to one's humanistic healer role is increasingly more difficult as the physician's role has expanded beyond providing knowledge and prescribing treatment plans. Modern health care advancements, the increased availability and marketing of most diagnostic tests and treatments, the easy availability of high-quality Internet-based medical knowledge, and the rise of the consumer culture also contribute to the potential loss of patient-centeredness (Bombeke et al. 2010; Stern et al. 2008).

Furthermore, the growing pressures in the medical system for higher efficiency and productivity threaten the physician's ability to maintain a good attitude and work ethic while providing humanistic health care.

Physicians have increasingly limited time with their patients as the demands for patient volume and revenue rise. Increasingly, physicians devote more time in the physician-patient encounter to clerical tasks such as typing in medical orders and appropriate diagnostic codes, as well as completing other tasks within electronic health records required to obtain reimbursement. Many physicians feel rushed and stressed by time constraints, which can adversely affect their attitudes and work ethic. The old Irish proverb "Quick and well-done do not agree" is especially true in medical care. Haste is not compatible with a good attitude and work ethic in the practice of medicine because it negatively affects essential elements such as focused observation, attentive listening, and the expression of humanistic qualities such as empathy and compassion (Bombeke et al. 2010). Thus, in the realm of medical education, one can easily understand how these challenges and pressures can adversely affect a physician's attitude, work ethic, and ability to act as a positive role model for their learners and to provide effective teaching.

Conceptual Framework

Academic medical institutions are complex dynamic systems with webs of relationships (W. L. Miller et al. 1998). Learning opportunities in clinical medicine follow a series of socially negotiated interactions within and between individuals and their environment (McLellan et al. 2015). Thus, "medical practice is more the maintenance of a network of human relationships than the application of scientific knowledge" (Olthuis and Dekkers 2003, p. 929). We found it helpful to consider complexity theory to develop our own framework for promoting a good attitude and work ethic within the complex system of health care and medical education (Rickles et al. 2007).

The health care system relies on multidisciplinary interactions for the provision of competent patient care and the delivery of effective medical education. Furthermore, the health care team is comprised of highly variable team members (learners, patients, teachers, clinicians, allied health professionals, administrators, and others) who assemble ad hoc depending on their skill, expertise, clinical duty, and schedule. The work environment of these team members is also highly variable because patients' illnesses and care do not follow a standardized schedule. Thus, the work and learning environment is a complex system. Additionally, institutional history and culture influence the health care systems. Thus, the health care environment is a dynamic, flexible, and adaptable complex system that does not follow a linear process where "x" results in "y." Instead, this system can transform unpredictably over time in response to the implementation of even small changes from team members (Caffrey et al. 2016; McLellan et al. 2015; Rickles et al. 2007; Jorm et al. 2016).

Complexity theory, which originated in the fields of mathematics and chaos theory (Rickles et al. 2007), is an approach to studying complex systems that focuses "on the interactions between system components" (Jorm et al. 2016, p. 2). Applying complexity theory to medical education suggests that the components or team members (learners, patients, teachers, clinicians, allied health professionals, administrators, and others) "act, react and adapt" in accordance with their unique perspectives and experiences (Caffrey et al. 2016). Therefore, when trying to understand and promote good attitude and work ethic in academic medical institutions, recognition of the complexity of the educational and clinical health care system is essential.

We applied complexity theory to promoting a good attitude and work ethic in medical education by first recognizing that faculty need to build a supportive learning and work environment (Figure 3). This environment creates an atmosphere where learners and faculty can discuss their own beliefs, weaknesses, doubts and mistakes (L. G. Cohen and Sherif 2014). Faculty should greet learners with enthusiasm each day and, whenever possible, find something positive to say about them. They should share stories or other aspects of their personal lives with learners, talking briefly about a good movie, an inspiring book, hobbies, interesting travels, or favorite family activities (Bombeke et al. 2010). This makes the learners more comfortable in sharing their own experiences, whether they are positive or negative.

Faculty should make a conscientious effort to promote confidence among learners by praising them for their progress, talents, and diligent work. They should also promote activities that support learners working collaboratively to foster interpersonal interactions and teamwork. Jorm et al. (2016) used complexity theory to develop a large-scale interprofessional learning activity—the Health Collaboration Challenge—using case studies to understand how all the various health professional team members contribute to the care of a medically complex patient. They included learners from multiple disciplines (radiology, exercise physiology,

Supportive Learning and Work Environment

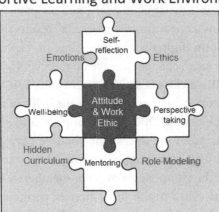

Figure 3. Conceptual framework of factors influencing attitude and work ethic of health professionals. Figure by authors.

medicine, nursing, occupational therapy, pharmacy, physical therapy, and speech therapy) who actively participated in developing a plan of care for each case. They designed their learning activity using Freeth et al.'s (2005) definition of an interprofessional learning activity, "learning arising from interaction between members of two or more professions" (p. 18) to prepare them for "interprofessional practice" (Jorm et al. 2016). The learners overwhelmingly recognized how health professional team members contribute to patient care, and described "negotiation, collaboration and creation of new collective knowledge" (Jorm et al. 2016 p. 1). This process provides the learners with practice opportunities to deal with the complex and dynamic health care system that they will be working in.

To promote a good attitude and work ethic, institutions and health care systems can provide training programs for their faculty and staff that include modules in hospitality, teamwork, communication, professionalism, responsibility, self-awareness, and physician-patient communication (Mueller 2009; UF College of Medicine 2014; Van Mook et al. 2009). Additionally, institutions can reinforce their commitment to promoting professionalism, including a positive attitude and work ethic, across the multiple disciplines by bolstering the health care professionals' ability to recognize and maintain humanistic attributes with the use of 360-degree peer evaluations (Joshi et al. 2004; Stark et al. 2008). These strategies help create a warm and welcoming atmosphere that is conducive to optimal learning and academic growth nested within the complex health care system.

Key Components for Promoting and Sustaining a Good Attitude and Work Ethic

Four key components within the complex milieu of a supportive learning and work environment are integral for promoting and sustaining a good attitude and work ethic.

1.Recognize the importance of emotions in patient care

Faculty can train learners to recognize, acknowledge, and reflect on emotions that surface during interactions with patients (Bombeke et al. 2010). Bombeke et al. note that learners can become "overwhelmed by suffering" (2010), especially when confronted with emotions and life experiences that they had not previously experienced. Learners can benefit from formal opportunities in various settings to learn how to recognize and respond to their patients' emotional states in a therapeutic fashion. For example, case studies, small groups, standardized patient exercises, group learning activities, and clinical rotations are possible formats and settings that faculty can utilize (L. G. Cohen and Sherif 2014). Learners need exposure to varying clinical scenarios, including those associated with profoundly positive emotions commonly experienced in the medical practice. Failure to address or inadequately addressing difficult situations or unpleasant emotions can traumatize learners (Kumagai et al. 2017). As Kumagai and colleagues note, the objective for the faculty is not to avoid distress, but to provide an environment that allows for respectful dialogue (Kumagai et al. 2017). Thus, faculty can help prepare learners to "negotiate meaning, and resolve epistemological differences" (Spelt et al. 2009, p. 373) with others they may not know well (Jorm et al. 2016). This preparation is "crucial to learners' personal and professional moral development" (Kumagai et al. 2017, p. 318), and faculty can serve as the learners' guide. By acknowledging and discussing the spectrum of emotional responses garnered from medical encounters, faculty can convey to their learners that emotions matter and are inseparable from reason and problem solving in medical care.

2. Introduce formal ethics teaching

Whenever possible, teaching objectives should include links to formal ethics teaching. For example, when faculty discuss end-of-life care with a patient or their family, they should prompt learners to reflect on the concept of death, respect for the patient's preferences, and dignity in death (Olthuis and Dekkers 2003). Similarly, when teaching how to perform a history and physical exam, there is an opportunity for faculty to teach the principles of truthfulness, respect for patients, confidentiality, and shared decision making (Siegler 2001). Additionally, faculty need to recognize that some learners may need to receive training in etiquette-based communication that includes introducing yourself and explaining your role, as well as attentive listening (Block et al. 2013). Faculty may need to instruct learners to be truthful about their student status and to ask for the patients' permission to participate in their care, as it is a privilege.

There is no consensus for the best approach for teaching of ethics in medical education. Hafferty and Franks (1994) propose an environment integrating ethical principles into the learners' professional identity, combining "elements of knowledge with elements of identity" (Hafferty and Franks 1994, p. 867). This approach is distinct from the method of teaching the basic sciences where the knowledge of topic exists independently from the learner. Thus, all faculty need to identify and convey ethical issues they encounter to their learners via their words and behavior (Hafferty and Franks 1994).

3. Act as positive role models in attitude and work ethic

As role models, faculty have a strong influence in shaping their learners' professional identity (Bombeke et al. 2010; Burgess et al. 2015; Kenny et al. 2003). Therefore, faculty should act as role models by explicitly demonstrating a good attitude and work ethic to build respectful connections with patients, family members, and the medical team. As positive role models, faculty should display enthusiasm, dedication, humility, tolerance, honesty, and politeness. They should demonstrate the behaviors of attentive listening, making eye contact, adjusting tone of voice, and altering the rate of speech (Bombeke et al. 2010). Additionally, faculty should not be dismissive of patients' emotions, but rather they should provide appropriate time for patients to express their emotions and respond to them empathically. Exemplary role models acknowledge patients' affective and emotional responses (L. G. Cohen and Sherif 2014). Other key characteristics are punctuality and maintaining respectful interactions with other professionals. Faculty should strive to increase their conscious awareness of role modeling, which can have a strong impact on their learners' development of a good attitude and work ethic (S. R. Cruess et al. 2008; Mueller 2009).

4. Address the hidden curriculum

The hidden curriculum can be a silent threat to the development of a good attitude and work ethic (Hafferty and Franks 1994). The hidden curriculum has a "powerful influence on learners and is largely delivered by role models" (Mueller 2009, p. 137). Faculty need to be cognizant that learners may be more inclined to incorporate the negative behaviors conveyed by the hidden curriculum, despite the explicit curriculum's emphasis on humanistic practices in medical care. For example, when learners observe that faculty do not regularly introduce themselves to their patients, or they fail to take time to listen to their patients' stories or to acknowledge their emotions, they may deduce that these negative behaviors are acceptable and likely necessary for optimal work efficiency.

In addition to the hidden curriculum, Nelson et al. (1992) describe the "null curriculum": the educational material intentionally left out. Learners assume that left-out material is unimportant. For example, if communication or physician-patient relations are not included in the preclinical years, learners may not value these topics as worthy of investing their time in. Woloschuk et al. (2004) posit this omission may partially explain why learners' scores, as assessed in their study by the Attitudes Toward Social Issues in Medicine scale, decreased as they went from the preclinical to the clinical years. Thus, faculty should try to explicitly identify and discuss the detrimental effects of the hidden and null curricula with learners. This effort will help them adhere to the practice of the humanistic behaviors taught in the explicit curriculum (L. G. Cohen and Sherif 2014; Jaye et al. 2005).

Tools to Aid in Promoting and Sustaining a Good Attitude and Work Ethic among Learners

1. Self-reflection

The self-reflection method helps learners to acquire a better appreciation of their emotional responses, values, and attitudes, which arise during or after a medical encounter. By means of the self-reflection method, learners can obtain the skills to become more reflective, self-conscious, and interpersonally conscious during clinical encounters (Burks and Kobus 2012). Although reflecting on experiences does not sound like a difficult task, most experts recommend formal training and practice in self-reflection for obtaining optimal results (Stern et al. 2008). We advise learners to maintain journals describing clinical situations that show professionalism or lack thereof. They should meet periodically with their faculty preceptor to go over these clinical experiences. The faculty's goal is for learners to become more conscious of what has happened during a specific encounter. Learners should analyze their assumptions and responses. In addition, we encourage them to investigate what others with different points of view might bring to the same experience. Finally, learners should strive to integrate this new knowledge into their future interactions (Stern et al. 2008).

Examples of two medical students' self-reflection narratives follow. One medical student wrote:

> The medical team was rounding and entered the patient's room. There were eight team members in the room. Our team discussed the patient's case, examined him and agreed on a treatment plan for the day. The patient was older and hard of hearing but the team members left without making sure he understood the plan for his care or if he had any questions. I felt disappointed by the team's lack of communication skills and respect for this patient. I decided to stay at the patient's bedside and carefully explain the plan of care to him after everyone else had left the room.

Another medical student wrote:

> I was asked to shadow my preceptor who was examining an older woman. . . . Following the physical examination, the woman had a

few questions about health maintenance. She was trying to explain why she would not receive vaccines but my attending kept on interrupting her before she made her points. The attending constantly looked toward the computer screen and never made any eye contact with the patient. This appeared cold and unprofessional.

2. Perspective taking

When utilizing this method, the learner takes the point of view of another person and gains improved insight of what it is like to be in the other person's situation. This exercise enhances empathy and allows medical professionals to become more understanding of certain behaviors displayed by their patients or coworkers (Burks and Kobus 2012). We believe medical educators should encourage their learners to practice perspective taking during interpersonal interactions at work. The examples below illustrate situations in which the employment of perspective taking can be an effective means of making us more empathetic and better prepared to manage the challenging behaviors in question. Therefore, perspective taking can contribute to improving our attitude and work ethic toward patients and coworkers.

When can we use perspective taking?

A patient refuses to have a screening colonoscopy because his sister had a bowel perforation as a complication from this procedure.

Perspective taking in this situation allows us to recognize the patient's concern for a procedure-related complication. After explaining the risks versus benefits of the procedure, we can then take into account the patient's preference and offer stool test screening.

A patient on a limited income is nonadherent to his medical therapy due to his inability to afford medications.

Perspective taking in this case allows us to recognize our bias in labeling the patient as nonadherent based on their financial situation. After recognizing this, we can then work with the patient's pharmacy to find lower cost alternatives for this patient.

A 30-year-old woman who is in the last stages of terminal cancer is hesitant to sign a Do Not Resuscitate form because she is the primary caregiver of small children.

Perspective taking in this case informs us of the patient's rationale for a decision that at first seems to indicate denial of the severity of her illness. We can discuss possible options and other avenues potentially available that will respect her preferences.

3. Mentoring

Mentoring can be a powerful method for helping learners to acquire solid principles of professionalism and thereby improve their attitude and work ethic. Due to the increasing volume of medical knowledge and practice changes in medicine, learners can no longer solely rely on learning via didactic lectures and experiential learning. The value of mentoring in medical education is crucial to advancing the learner's development (Platz and Hyman 2013). Effective mentors facilitate discussions about work experiences and promote the practice of self-reflection and perspective taking (Stern et al. 2008). Mentors can be instrumental in providing psychological support during challenging work situations. They promote the formation of a positive interpersonal code of conduct and help etch the invaluable traits of good attitude and work ethic into a novice health care professional's skill set. Mentors share their unique knowledge gained from personal experience; academic textbooks do not contain this information. Furthermore, mentors can openly discuss the negative and positive effects of the hidden curriculum and they can teach how to practice the art of medicine (Hafferty and Franks 1994).

For example, a first-year surgical resident comes in for his semiannual meeting with his mentor. The mentor greets him warmly and they sit down to discuss the resident's experience and to review his evaluations. The resident is pleased overall but admits to being under a lot of stress. He relates his stress to being constantly under time constraints and to his fear of making mistakes during surgical procedures. The mentor reviews his evaluations and commends him for his excellent scores in medical knowledge and teaching. The mentor also points out to the resident his below-average scores in medical professionalism. The resident appears shocked and quite uncomfortable with the news. On further review, his below-average grades in professionalism came mostly from nurses. The mentor has many years of experience in this medical institution and is able to relate the resident's poor score in humanistic attributes to negative effects of the hidden curriculum. The mentor discusses the institution's culture of poor rapport between nurses and surgical residents. Surgical residents are always under stress, and nurses perceive them as impatient and rude. The mentor suggests challenging the institutional culture by asking the resident to make a conscious effort to respond promptly to nurses and treat them with more respect. The mentor explains how this would improve the resident's work atmosphere and result in better patient care. In addition, it would certainly have a positive impact in his future evaluations.

4. Promoting well-being

The demands of increasing knowledge and clinical workload, as well the detrimental effects of the hidden curriculum, can lead to burnout. Faculty need to promote well-being to counterbalance the factors in medical education that threaten the healer role of the physician and negatively affect attitude and work ethic (Novack et al. 1999). Well-being is the sense of happiness and positive attitude that stems from feeling fulfilled and content (Diener 2000). Promoting well-being requires that learners become aware of their own emotions, experiences, and perceptions (Novack et al. 1997), which allows them to grow and develop their physician healer role (Novack et al. 1999).

Novack et al. (1999 p. 517) state that the overall goals for medical education should ensure that learners "understand how their personal histories, personal lives, as well as their values, attitudes and biases" affect patient care, and how learners can "care for themselves physically and emotionally" (Novack et al. 1999 p. 518). Mechanisms for developing self-awareness and well-being include "support groups, Balint groups, literature discussions, family-of-origin groups, discussions of meaningful experiences in medicine," as well as confidential counseling (Novack et al. 1999, p. 518). Faculty may need additional training and development themselves to effectively role-model and promote well-being to their learners.

Final Thoughts

Interactions consistently displaying a good attitude and work ethic are the most effective way of building strong interpersonal work relationships. We need more research to identify the most efficient methods to foster a culture of good attitude and work ethic, as well as to measure the attitudes of learners. Then we can triangulate these measurements with burnout scales and other scales for emotional well-being.

Questions for Future Research

How do we determine the value of interventions in training medical teams to have a good attitude and work ethic at the beginning of an inpatient or outpatient rotation?

How do we measure the value of offering faculty development courses for mentors on how to teach having a good attitude and work ethic to their learners?

What is the best format for delivering institution-wide training programs on having a good attitude and work ethic?

How does a good attitude and work ethic relate to burnout?

References

Abelson, J., Maxwell, P. H., and Maxwell, R. J. (1997). Do professions have a future? *BMJ* 315(7105): 382–382. doi: 10.1136/bmj.315.7105.382.

ABIM Foundation, American Board of Internal Medicine, ACP-ASIM Foundation (American College of Physicians-American Society of Internal Medicine), and European Federation of Internal Medicine. (2002). Medical professionalism in the new millennium: A physician charter. *Annals of Internal Medicine* 136(3): 243–246. doi: 10.7326/0003-4819-136-3-200202050-00012.

Arnold, L., and Stern, D. T. (2006). What is medical professionalism? In D. T. Stern (Ed.): *Measuring medical professionalism* (pp. 15–37) Oxford University Press.

Birden, H., Glass, N., Wilson, I., Harrison, M., Usherwood, T., and Nass, D. (2014). Defining professionalism in medical education: A systematic review. *Medical Teacher* 36(1): 47–61. doi: 10.3109/0142159x.2014.850154.

Block, L., Hutzler, L., Habicht, R., Wu, A. W., Desai, S. V., Novello Silva, K., . . . Feldman, L. (2013). Do internal medicine interns practice etiquette-based communication? A critical look at the inpatient encounter. *Journal of Hospital Medicine* 8(11): 631–634. doi: 10.1002/jhm.2092.

Blumenthal, D. (1994). The vital role of professionalism in health care reform. *Health Affairs*, 13(1): 252–256. doi: 10.1377/hlthaff.13.1.252.

Bombeke, K., Symons, L., Debaene, L., Winter, B. D., Schol, S., and Van Royen, P. (2010). Help, I'm losing patient-centredness! Experiences of medical students and their teachers. *Medical Education* 44(7): 662–673. doi: 10.1111/j.1365-2923.2010.03627.x.

Brody, H., and Doukas, D. (2014). Professionalism: A framework to guide medical education. *Medical Education* 48(10): 980–987. doi: 10.1111/medu.12520.

Burgess, A., Oates, K., and Goulston, K. (2015). Role modelling in medical education: The importance of teaching skills. *Clinical Teacher* 13(2): 134–137. doi: 10.1111/tct.12397.

Burks, D. J., and Kobus, A. M. (2012). The legacy of altruism in health care: The promotion of empathy, prosociality and humanism. *Medical Education* 46(3): 317–325. doi: 10.1111/j.1365-2923.2011.04159.x.

Caffrey, L., Wolfe, C., and Mckevitt, C. (2016). Embedding research in health systems: Lessons from complexity theory. *Health Research Policy and Systems* 14(1): 54. doi: 10.1186/s12961-016-0128-x.

Charles, C., Gafni, A., and Whelan, T. (1997). Shared decision-making in the medical encounter: What does it mean? (or it takes at least two to tango). *Social Science and Medicine* 44(5): 681–692. doi: 10.1016/s0277-9536(96)00221-3.

Cohen, J. J. (2007). Viewpoint: Linking professionalism to humanism: What it means, why it matters. *Academic Medicine* 82(11): 1029–1032. doi: 10.1097/01.acm.0000285307.17430.74.

Cohen, L. G., and Sherif, Y. A. (2014). Twelve tips on teaching and learning humanism in medical education. *Medical Teacher* 36(8): 680–684. doi: 10.3109/0142159x.2014.916779.

Colgan, R. (2014). The virtuous physician. *Consultant* 54(8): 594–597.

Cruess, S. R., and Cruess, R. L. (1997). Professionalism must be taught. *BMJ* 315(7123): 1674–1677. doi: 10.1136/bmj.315.7123.1674.

Cruess, R. L., and Cruess, S. R. (1997). Teaching medicine as a profession in the service of healing. *Academic Medicine* 72(11): 941–952. doi: 10.1097/00001888-199711000-00009.

Cruess, R. L., Cruess, S. R., and Johnston, S. E. (1999). Renewing professionalism: An opportunity for medicine. *Academic Medicine* 74(8): 878–884. doi: 10.1097/00001888-199908000-00010.

Cruess, S. R., Cruess, R. L., and Steinert, Y. (2008). Role modelling—making the most of a powerful teaching strategy. *BMJ* 336(7646): 718–721. doi: 10.1136/bmj.39503.757847.be.

Diener, E. (2000). Subjective well-being: The science of happiness and a proposal for a national index. *American Psychologist* 55(1): 34–43. doi: 10.1037//0003-066x.55.1.34.

Epstein, R. M. (1999). Mindful practice. *JAMA*, 282(9): 833–839. doi: 10.1001/jama.282.9.833.

Frankford, D. M., Patterson, M. A., and Konrad, T. R. (2000). Transforming practice organizations to foster lifelong learning and commitment to medical professionalism. *Academic Medicine* 75(7): 708–717. doi: 10.1097/00001888-200007000-00012.

Freeth, D., Hammick, M., Reeves, S., Koppel, I., and Barr, H. (2005). *Effective interprofessional education: Development, delivery and evaluation.* John Wiley Sons.

Freidson, E. (1988). *Professional powers: A study of the institutionalization of formal knowledge*. Chicago: University of Chicago Press.

Gerteis, M., Edgman-Levitan, S., Daley, J., and Delbanco, T. L. (eds.). (1993). *Through the patient's eyes: Understanding and promoting patient-centered care*. San Francisco: Jossey-Bass.

Ginsburg, S., Regehr, G., Hatala, R., Mcnaughton, N., Frohna, A., Hodges, B., . . . Stern, D. (2000). Context, conflict, and resolution: A new conceptual framework for evaluating professionalism. *Academic Medicine* 75(10, Supplement): S6–S11. doi: 10.1097/00001888-200010001-00003.

Hafferty, F. W., and Franks, R. (1994). The hidden curriculum, ethics teaching, and the structure of medical education. *Academic Medicine* 69(11): 861–871. doi: 10.109 7/00001888-199411000-00001.

Haug, M. R. (1972). Deprofessionalization: An alternate hypothesis for the future. *Sociological Review* 20(S1): 195–211. doi: 10.1111/j.1467-954x.1972.tb03217.x.

Hilton, S., and Southgate, L. (2007). Professionalism in medical education. *Teaching and Teacher Education* 23(3): 265–279. doi: 10.1016/j.tate.2006.12.024.

Irvine, D. (1997). The performance of doctors. I: Professionalism and self regulation in a changing world. *BMJ* 314(7093): 1540. doi: 10.1136/bmj.314.7093.1540.

Jaye, C., Egan, T., and Parker, S. (2005). Learning to be a doctor: Medical educators talk about the hidden curriculum in medical education. *Focus on Health Professional Education: A Multi-Disciplinary Journal* 7(2): 1–17.

Jorm, C., Nisbet, G., Roberts, C., Gordon, C., Gentilcore, S., and Chen, T. F. (2016). Using complexity theory to develop a student-directed interprofessional learning activity for 1220 healthcare students. *BMC Medical Education* 16(1): 199. doi: 10.1186/s12909-016-0717-y.

Joshi, R., Ling, F. W., and Jaeger, J. (2004). Assessment of a 360-degree instrument to evaluate residents' competency in interpersonal and communication skills. *Academic Medicine* 79(5): 458–463. doi: 10.1097/00001888-200405000-00017.

Kelly, M. E., Fenlon, N. P. and Murphy, A. W. (2002). An approach to the education about, and the assessment of, attitudes in undergraduate medical education. *Irish Journal of Medical Science* 171(4): 206–210. doi: 10.1007/BF03170282.

Kenny, N. P., Mann, K. V., and Macleod, H. (2003). Role modeling in physicians' professional formation: Reconsidering an essential but untapped educational strategy. *Academic Medicine* 78(12): 1203–1210. doi: 10.1097/00001888-200312000-00002.

Kumagai, A. K., Jackson, B., and Razack, S. (2017). Cutting close to the bone: Student trauma, free speech, and institutional responsibility in medical education. *Academic Medicine* 92(3): 318–323. doi: 10.1097/acm.0000000000001425.

McLellan, L., Yardley, S., Norris, B., de Bruin, A., Tully, M. P., and Dornan, T. (2015). Preparing to prescribe: How do clerkship students learn in the midst of complexity? *Advances in Health Sciences Education* 20(5): 1339–1354. doi: 10.1007/s10459-015-9606-0.

Mead, N., and Bower, P. (2000). Patient-centredness: A conceptual framework and review of the empirical literature. *Social Science and Medicine* 51(7): 1087–1110. doi: 10.1016/s0277-9536(00)00098-8.

Mechanic, D. (1985). Public perceptions of medicine. *New England Journal of Medicine* 312(3): 181–183. doi: 10.1056/nejm198501173120312.

Miller, M. J., Woehr, D. J., and Hudspeth, N. (2001). The meaning and measurement of work ethic: Construction and initial validation of a multidimensional inventory. *Journal of Vocational Behavior* 59, 1–39. doi: 10.1006/jvbe.2001.1838.

Miller, W. L., Crabtree, B. F., McDaniel, R., and Stange, K. C. (1998). Understanding change in primary care practice using complexity theory. *Journal of Family Practice* 46(5): 369–376.

Mueller, P. S. (2009). Incorporating professionalism into medical education: The Mayo Clinic experience. *Keio Journal of Medicine* 58(3): 133–143. doi: 10.2302/kjm.58.133.

Nelson, M., Jacobs, C., and Cuban, L. (1992). Concepts of curriculum. *Teaching and Learning in Medicine, 4*(4): 202–205. doi: 10.1080/10401339209539565.

Newble, D. I. (1992). Assessing clinical competence at the undergraduate level. *Medical Education* 26(6): 503–511. doi: 10.1111/j.1365–2923.1992.tb00213.x.

Novack, D. H., Epstein, R. M., and Paulsen, R. H. (1999). Toward creating physician-healers: Fostering medical students' self-awareness, personal growth, and well-being. *Academic Medicine* 74(5): 516–520. doi: 10.1097/00001888–199905000–00017.

Novack, D. H., Suchman, A. L., Clark, W., Epstein, R. M., Najberg, E., and Kaplan, C. (1997). Calibrating the physician: Personal awareness and effective patient care. Working Group on Promoting Physician Personal Awareness, American Academy on Physician and Patient. *JAMA* 278(6): 502–509. doi: 10.1001/jama.278.6.502.

Olthuis, G., and Dekkers, W. (2003). Medical education, palliative care and moral attitude: Some objectives and future perspectives. *Medical Education* 37(10): 928–933. doi: 10.1046/j.1365–2923.2003.01635.x.

Platz, J., and Hyman, N. (2013). Mentorship. *Clinics in Colon and Rectal Surgery* 26(04): 218–223. doi: 10.1055/s-0033–1356720.

Porter, R. (1997). *The greatest benefit to mankind: A medical history of humanity.* New York: Norton.

Rickles, D., Hawe, P., and Shiell, A. (2007, 11). A simple guide to chaos and complexity. *Journal of Epidemiology and Community Health* 61(11): 933–937. doi: 10.1136/jech.2006.054254.

Rothman, D. J. (2000). Medical professionalism—Focusing on the real issues. *New England Journal of Medicine* 343(10): 739–740. *342*(17): 1284–1286. doi: 10.1056/nejm 200009073431014.

Siegler, M. (2001). Lessons from 30 Years of teaching clinical ethics. *Virtual Mentor* 3(10). doi: 10.1001/virtualmentor.2001.3.10.medu1–0110.

Sohl, P., and Bassford, H. (1986). Codes of medical ethics: Traditional foundations and contemporary practice. *Social Science & Medicine* 22(11): 1175–1179. doi: 10.1016/0277–9536(86)90184-x.

Spelt, E. J., Biemans, H. J., Tobi, H., Luning, P. A., and Mulder, M. (2009). Teaching and learning in interdisciplinary higher education: A systematic review. *Educational Psychology Review* 21(4): 365. doi: 10.1007/s10648–009–9113-z.

Stark, R., Korenstein, D., and Karani, R. (2008). Impact of a 360-degree professionalism assessment on faculty comfort and skills in feedback delivery. *Journal of General Internal Medicine* 23(7): 969–972. doi: 10.1007/s11606-008-0586-0.

Stern, D. T., Cohen, J. J., Bruder, A., Packer, B., and Sole, A. (2008). Teaching humanism. *Perspectives in biology and medicine* 51(4): 495–507. doi: 10.1353/pbm.0.0059.

Swick, H. M. (2000, 06). Toward a normative definition of medical professionalism. *Academic Medicine* 75(6): 612–616. doi: 10.1097/00001888-200006000-00010.

Swick, H. M., Szenas, P., Danoff, D., and Whitcomb, M. E. (1999, 09). Teaching professionalism in undergraduate medical education. *JAMA* 282(9): 830–832. doi: 10.1001/jama.282.9.830.

University of Florida (UF) College of Medicine. (2014). *Faculty Matters*. May. Hospitality and service training to begin. Retrieved from https://com-faculty-affairs.sites.medinfo.ufl.edu/files/2014/05/May2014.pdf.

Van Mook, W. N., de Grave, W. S., van Luijk, S. J., O'Sullivan, H., Wass, V., Schuwirth, L. W., and van der Vleuten, C. P. (2009, July). Training and learning professionalism in the medical school curriculum: Current considerations. *European Journal of Internal Medicine* 20(4). doi: 10.1016/j.ejim.2008.12.006.

Woloschuk, W., Harasym, P. H., and Temple, W. (2004). Attitude change during medical school: A cohort study. *Medical Education* 38(5): 522–534. doi: 10.1046/j.1365-2929.2004.01820.x.

4

Professional Identity Formation

MELANIE GROSS HAGEN, NEAL HOLLAND, AND LYNN MONROUXE[1]

Non nobis solum nati sumus—We are not born for ourselves alone.
Cicero

In this chapter a review of literature on paradigms related to professional identity formation (PIF), specifically social identity theory, is provided. We use a vignette to guide the reader through the process that learners experience during the transformation from layperson to physician. Additionally, we provide guidelines for educators to help facilitate the process of PIF in learners during transition periods.

Objectives

Review concepts of identity formation in adults.
Define the concept of professional identity.
Contrast professionalism with professional identity.
Apply ideas in social identity theory to professional identity formation in medical trainees.

Transition from Medical School to Internship

Jessica is an Asian American completing her fourth year of medicine at a medical school in the United States. It is match day, the day that graduating seniors find out where they have been placed to do their residency training. She has just received notification that she matched at her top choice program in internal medicine in the northeastern U.S.

---

1   Melanie Gross Hagen, M.D., F.A.C.P., University of Florida College of Medicine, Gainesville, FL.
Neal Holland, D.O., University of Florida College of Medicine, Gainesville, FL.
Lynn Monrouxe, Ph.D., Chang Gung Memorial Hospital, Taoyuan City 333, Taiwan (R.O.C.).

"Yes, I made it," she thinks. Then, she sits down and contemplates, "Am I ready for this?"

Transition from Resident to Attending

Jessica just received a call offering her a job as an attending physician at an academic medical center in the city in which she finished her training. She accepts the job because it offers the combination of inpatient and outpatient responsibilities, benefits, and salary that she had been looking for. "I am so excited to finally have finished my training. But, now I will be the one ultimately responsible for patient care." She feels a sudden sense of vulnerability.

Jessica starts work at her new position. Her role includes treating patients in an ambulatory care practice and as a hospital teaching attending physician. She shares some concerns with a friend: "I miss the sense of teamwork I felt during residency. It is like I am working in a vacuum, just the patients and I."

Multiple Identities

Three years later Jessica is nine months pregnant and ready to deliver her baby any day.

"I wonder if I will be able to give my baby all the attention she needs. In the prenatal classes I attend, all the mothers are stay-at-home-moms, who tell me that they made the decision to stay home to take care of their children themselves. The one mom who is working is always looking stressed!"

Professional identify formation (PIF) refers to a process through which a learner transforms into a health care professional. PIF is an "integration of personal values, morals, and attributes with the norms of the profession" (Wilson et al. 2013). An individual learns the knowledge and skills necessary to administer medical care and begins to envision him- or herself as a health care professional. This chapter introduces the concept of PIF to the medical educator. The development of a professional identity happens "simultaneously at two levels: 1) at the level of the individual, which involves the psychological development of the person and 2) at the collective level, which involves the socialization of the person into appropriate roles and forms of participation in the community's work" (Jarvis-Selinger et al. 2012, p. 1185). Much of this socialization arises within the medical educator-learner relationship (Monrouxe and Rees 2017). In this chapter, we contrast PIF with other concepts of professionalism. Using the social identity theory framework, we explain how both psychological and sociological factors influence professional identity formation.

Defining Professionalism

The difference between professionalism and the development of professional identity is not always clear. The traditional conception of professionalism is virtue-based; it assumes learners automatically acquire "values and beliefs" during training (R. L. Cruess and Cruess 2016b). Older characterizations define professionalism according to the qualities that drive physicians and result in behaviors beneficial to others. These qualities include service to others, competency, scholarship, communication, ethical and legal understanding, application of excellence, humanism, accountability, and altruism (R. L. Cruess and Cruess 2016b). Recently, the American Board of Medical Specialties (ABMS) described professionalism as when practitioners strive to:

> acquire, maintain and advance: 1) an ethical value system grounded in the conviction that the medical profession exists to serve patients' and the public's interests, and not merely the self-interests of practitioners; 2) the knowledge and technical skills necessary for good medical practice; and 3) the interpersonal skills necessary to work together with patients, eliciting goals and values to direct the proper use of the profession's specialized knowledge and skills, sometimes referred to as the "art" of medicine. (ABMS Board of Directors 2012, p. 1)

During the mid- to late 20th century, medical educators began to fear that natural observation and emulation of physician role models was insufficient to instill the values and beliefs of the medical profession set forth in the Hippocratic Oath (R. L. Cruess and Cruess 2016b). Some physicians put their own needs ahead of those of patients, and learners did not always have the ability or desire to select only good role models to emulate (R. L. Cruess and Cruess 2016b). These problems threatened the tradition of professionalism; consequently, concerned educators developed a move-ment to realign medical training to include explicit delineation of and training in professionalism (ABIM Foundation et al. 2002; Kirk 2007).

Clarifying the Difference between Professionalism and PIF

Professional identity is more than behaving professionally (Monrouxe et al. 2011). Clinicians and learners may act professionally in a social setting to gain approval. Conversely, learners may possess professional attitudes but act unprofessionally in response to social pressures (Rees and Knight 2007). Studying the way an individual develops, maintains, and expands a professional identity helps us to understand how learners adopt values and attitudes (Monrouxe 2009). Richard and Sylvia Cruess define profes-sional identity as "a representation of self, achieved in stages over time, during which the characteristics, values, and norms of the medical pro-fession are internalized, resulting in an individual, thinking, acting, and feeling like a physician" (R. L. Cruess et al. 2015, p. 1447). The core of pro-fessional identity comprises values including caring, compassion, com-mitment, confidentiality, honesty, and integrity (R. L. Cruess and Cruess 2016b). Professional identity achievement is the fifth level, "Is," of Miller's pyramid, a structured approach to assessment of medical competence (R. L. Cruess et al. 2016). A professional identity leads to internal regulation of ethical behavior as well as confidence and a professional demeanor (Monrouxe 2009).

The concept of professional identity highlights the difference between clinicians' *potential,* captured by definitions of professionalism, and their *actual* ability in the moment to adapt to change, incorporate new knowledge, and use continual performance feedback. In defining profes-sional identity, researchers and theorists incorporate interpersonal and complexity discourses (Monrouxe et al. 2011). This concept represents a step toward the goal of actually *being* a professional, characterized as an "interpersonal, complex activity," rather than simply *acting* professionally (Monrouxe et al. 2011, p. 588)

We can also contrast PIF with virtue-based and behavior-based profes-sionalism (Irby and Hamstra 2016). Virtue-based professionalism centers on an individual's moral character. The goal is to commit to a "set of values and actions guided by moral reasoning" (Irby and Hamstra 2016, p. 1607). In contrast, behavior-based professionalism focuses on demonstrating behaviors and reaching milestones and competencies. PIF, on the other hand, develops as the result of socialization into a community of practice, which aims to provide positive role models for students so that they are then alert to the existence of negative role models when they see them (Irby and Hamstra 2016). To illustrate the relevance of PIF for a typical learner, recall the vignette at the start of the chapter, which illustrates critical transition points in the life of Jessica, a doctor in training.

Models of Identity Formation

The identity of a learner, viewed from an individual or societal level, is where a person socializes into their role in the community (Monrouxe 2016). A coherent identity most commonly forms by adulthood, but is not static. An individual's identity may be affected by many factors and circumstances, including gender, race, social practices, institutional arrangements, and cultural ideologies. Additionally, individuals may belong to several groups with different identities that may or may not overlap. For example, in our case study, Jessica is a mother, a physician, and a Chinese-American. Multiple experiences impact any individual's identity, and at any given time, one identity may have a stronger influence than others (Tsouroufli et al. 2011).

While this chapter focuses on the social identity model and theory for PIF, there are several other robust models and theories that describe identity formation, including those by Erickson, Marcia, Berzonsky, and Kegan (Berzonsky 1989; Erikson 1994; Kegan 1982; Marcia 1993).

Conceptual Framework

Identity is realized through a dynamic process of identification by which individuals classify their place in the world as both individuals and members of collectives. (Goldie 2012, p. e641)

In this section, we discuss the theoretical basis of social identity theory, then explore how this theory actualizes in medical education settings. Social identity theory describes the ways in which we conceptualize ourselves as belonging to a group (Abrams and Hogg 1990). Social identity theory is one of the most "influential theories of group processes and intergroup relations worldwide" (Hornsey 2008, p. 205). The theory has reconceptualized our understanding of the individual's relationship to the group and "extended its reach well outside the confines of social psychology" (Hornsey 2008, p. 205). We can understand a wide variety of social phenomena using social identity theory (Brewer 2001), including: receptiveness to interprofessional feedback between nurses and physicians; education of police officers about transgender people; the effect of ethnic threat on neighborhood association involvement; and obstacles to teamwork among health care assistants who care for patients with dementia (Miles-Johnson 2015; Savelkoul et al. 2015; Schaik et al. 2016; Lloyd et al. 2011).

An individual's identity formation is influenced by how he or she is seen by others and how others react to him or her. Our membership to groups is critical to our identity and how we interact with others. Social psychologist Floyd Allport (1979), whose work gave rise to social identity theory, first published the term "in-group" in the 1950s to describe the group with which an individual identifies. Those who do not belong to our group are part of the "out-group," a term coined by Tajfel and Turner (Tajfel 2010).

It is in this focus on the individual's relationship to the group that social identity theory differs from the principal alternative theory, sociocultural theory (Helmich and Dornan 2012). The sociocultural model is concerned with "the continuous negotiation of meaning and identity in interaction with other individuals that takes place in (socio-cultural) communities of practice" (Helmich and Dornan 2012, p. 132). Social identity theory, however, "considers group processes as something distinct from interpersonal interactions, but grounded firmly in individual cognition" (Burford 2012, p. 144). Thus, while the sociocultural approach examines interactions between people relating as independent individuals, social identity theory regards people as representatives of their groups (Hornsey 2008).

Individuals adopt a group identity through a process of self-categorization. This process is an example of the human cognitive pattern of organizing stimuli into categories. In this case, the tendency to categorize is motivated by self-interest (Burford 2012). Through self-categorization, an individual adopts a "'positive distinctiveness' on a valued dimension for one's own group (the 'in-group') compared to other groups (the 'out-groups')" (Burford 2012, p. 144). Thus, it is important not only which group one belongs to, but which group one does *not* belong to (Burford

2012). Members of a group have a positive bias toward others in their group compared to those outside their group. We also tend to conceive of our own group in a manner that highlights the differences between our group and other groups (Hogg and Reid 2006). As described by Hornsey (2008), we have the tendency to focus on similarities within our group members, tending to identify ourselves as like others in the group while enhancing our differences from other groups. This can be summarized as "we are all pretty much the same, and we are different from the other guys."

Founding social identity theorists such as Tajfel and Turner posit that the motivation for the competition between groups is the desire for a positive and secure self-image (Hornsey 2008). Logically, people want to think of their own group as the *best* group (Hornsey 2008). Previously, researchers believed the prime motivation for group behavior was self-esteem (Turner et al. 1994). More recently, however, the desire for uniqueness and self-definition has superseded self-esteem as the primary ascribed motivation for group behavior (Hornsey 2008). Thus, studies of group behavior are now more likely to focus on the desire to be distinct (Hornsey 2008).

According to social identity theory, individuals see group norms as prototypes that designate similarities within and differences between groups (Hogg and Reid 2006). When individuals categorize themselves and others, they internalize group norms as models for forming impressions, attitudes, feelings, and judgment for behavior (Hogg and Reid 2006). However, group norms are not static; they change based on the situation, depending on the strength of identification of each individual with alternate groups. The group maintains, expands and evolves its norms through communication about their group prototype (Hogg and Reid 2006).

Categorization into a group requires both that the group is *accessible* to an individual and that the individual is *fit* for the group (Burford 2012). These terms arise from cognitive theories about categorization. In this context, "accessibility" is defined as "the readiness with which a stimulus input with given properties will be coded or identified in terms of a category" (Turner et al. 1994, p. 289). A group's accessibility to an individual is a function of his or her "past experience, present expectations, and current motives, values goals and needs" (Turner et al. 1994, p. 289).

We each have our own perceptions of specific groups. According to social categorization theory, we use these perceptions to classify ourselves as being similar to or different from each group we encounter. We may identify with each group to a different degree. How we determine our fit is based on the activities that we participate in and whether we feel included in the group (Monrouxe 2016). The term "normative fit" describes the similarities we share with members of a group (Monrouxe 2016). Motivated by our desire for inclusion, we look for groups with which we can identify most strongly (Tajfel 2010).

In some situations, individuals may find that there is no group with which they easily identify. For example, moving to a more advanced level of training or a different phase in life may lead to a lack of available groups. In this case, individuals may identify themselves based on which group is the least different from them, a concept known as "comparative fit." The idea stems from the cognitive concept of categorization "in terms of the emergence of a focal category against contrasting background" (Turner et al. 1994, p. 289). In this method of categorization, individuals minimize the differences among members of a group in comparison to differences between groups. We identify with a group using a comparative fit when we cannot find a normative fit with a group.

The tendency to identify strongly with one group can pose challenges to society. Social identity theory predicts that the strength with which we identify with our own group is directly related to the extent to which we favor our group over the out-groups. As a result, the more secure we feel in our in-group, the more we cultivate our vision of our own group as exclusive and favorable compared to other groups. Nonetheless, different groups can work together in a positive manner if they share common goals in a supportive environment.

Application of Social Identity Theory to Medical Education

At the same time, individuals may have multiple identities available to them, which may be nested or hierarchical. The primary identity an individual uses at any one time depends on the context (Burford 2012). We must also remember that identity is not static; individuals' identities continue to change over their lives. Learners experience many transitions that influence the development of their professional identity. Identification within a social group can help individuals to handle stressful situations such as transitions (Haslam et al. 2005). Professional identities form as learners begin to feel part of an organization, such as premedical student associations, medical schools or hospital systems, professions (e.g., physicians, nurses, or administrators), and teams or departments (e.g., the emergency department, operating room, or primary care clinic).

Some trainees identify themselves as "premed" or "predoctors" as early as elementary school, a concept termed "anticipatory socialization" (Harvill 1981). Learners transition from premedical undergraduates to medical students, then to interns and residents, fellows, and finally attending physicians. Jarvis-Selinger et al. (2012) note that, rather than being a smooth and gradual course, these transitions occur in a discontinuous, stepwise process of movement from one stage to another in training. "Crises" or "abrupt discontinuities" characterize the transitions between stages (Jarvis-Selinger et al. 2012). A crisis arises when new events challenge an individual's current understanding of their professional identity (Jarvis-Selinger et al. 2012). Viewed through social identity theory, these transitions are stressful because the learner must cultivate a sense of fit with the new in-group.

After a transition, learners may take time to adjust to the new in-group. For example, medical students on a clinical team in an emergency room may at first identify most strongly with other medical students rather than physicians and other trained professionals. As the learners develop more responsibility and experience during training, they develop a fit for the physician group.

In addition to experience, context is also important in social identity formation. For example, in our case study, suppose Jessica was the only medical student in a rural emergency room. In this context, she might identify with the group of attending physicians or other Asian women on the team. For an individual who has completed medical training, the category of "doctor" may feel more accessible in the hospital or clinic than in a social environment (Burford 2012). For example, a physician parent at a children's athletic event may feel more like a parent than a physician if one of the children suffers a medical emergency.

The two most difficult and profound transitions for learners in medical training are the transition from student to physician and the transition from senior trainee to independent attending. During the transition from student to physician, learners take a leap in their responsibility and capacity. After being a junior member of the team, often acting more as a "shadow" than an effective professional, students leap over other members of the health care team they previously answered to, such as clerical staff, patient aids, nurses, therapists, and technicians. Now, instead of taking orders from others on the team, they lead the team. They have joined a new in-group of interns with the responsibility and power to give orders to the other members of the team, who may become their out-group. By spending many hours together, the interns may bond with one another over this new sense of responsibility. This intern peer group becomes a supportive family with a shared set of challenges and worries about competence. Another out-group for the interns may be the residents—trainees who have finished their internship—who interns see as more confident and more skilled than themselves. Interns are often isolated from peers in professions other than medicine, who have more time for social activities outside of the work environment. This serves to pull interns in closer to their in-group of colleagues and push them further from social contacts outside of medicine.

The transition from the learner to independent practitioner is also very challenging (Kumagai 2010), as it involves a leap in responsibility and a new leadership role. New attending physicians face novel tasks, roles, and settings (Kumagai 2010). A 2010 study of the transition in the Netherlands interviewed attending physicians soon after finishing residency and analyzed their experiences (Westerman et al. 2010). Using qualitative data, researchers made recommendations to ease this transition in the future, yet acknowledged that the struggle to meet new challenges led to personal growth for the research subjects. The researchers recommended better preparation in residency for the tasks required of attendings, and orientation programs to introduce new attendings to the workplace culture and organization. They also recommended peer groups in which new attendings can exchange experiences and use each other's feedback to model and practice skills (Westerman et al. 2010). This recommendation essentially advocates the formation of an in-group to cope with the transition.

Of course, each learner identifies with in-groups other than his or her profession. Learners have gender, cultural, and socioeconomic aspects to their identities, leading them to identify with other in-groups. For example, a learner may be a woman, a Cuban American, or a first-generation college graduate. Individuals may also be affected by experiences and circumstances that make them feel different than the norm (Tsouroufli et al. 2011). Learners' identities are a result of the *intersectionality* of their multiple experiences (Tsouroufli et al. 2011). This term describes the "set of unequal social relations" that "facilitated or constrained" an individual's sense of personal identity (Monrouxe 2015, p. 22). Monrouxe (2015) posits that by considering intersectionality in the study of PIF, we might achieve a more profound understanding of identity formation.

Let us explore how the theory of intersectionality sheds light on the complexity of social identity, and how social identity affects PIF. For example, a female intern may feel at a disadvantage compared to male colleagues, and may struggle to remain part of the in-group of interns when interacting with predominately female nurses. While the traditional doctor-nurse relationship carries some of the power differential of the traditional male-female relationship (Gjerberg and Kjølsrød 2001), the female interns and female nurses can relate to each other as women. They may share interests in fitness or travel. They may be of the same age and engaged in similar social activities, such as planning weddings or starting families. By identifying as young women, the young female doctors and nurses may develop their own in-group, to which the male interns do not belong. When the members of an individual's in-groups overlap, the individual has a simpler social identity. For example, if a Chinese-American female internist joins a play group with other Chinese-American internist mothers she will have simpler social identity than if she joined a group of mothers from other ethnic backgrounds who did not work outside the home. However, research shows that individuals with a more complex social identity structure are more likely to be inclusive of others and to tolerate those unlike themselves (Roccas and Brewer 2002).

Developing a professional identity can occasionally be troublesome for some learners (Goldie 2012). Some learners may sense that their class, gender, or ethnicity do not fit into the stereotypical image of a doctor and therefore have difficulty categorizing themselves as physicians. This struggle could be due to "failure to self-categorize as a doctor, or to identification with an inappropriate stereotype through lack of knowledge of their future role" (Burford 2012, p. 146).

Professional Identity and Behaviors on Diverse Teams

Despite explicit teaching, individuals may occasionally act unprofessionally. This conduct may seem surprising if we view professional behavior as static (R. L. Cruess et al. 2015). Yet learners may be imitating behaviors that they have seen by others in the doctor or trainee in-group. Using the concept of social identity helps us develop a new understanding of professional behavior and professional identity "by allowing norms to be viewed as dynamic and constructed in specific contexts" (Burford 2012, p. 146). Thus, as the norms of the in-group change in response to varying clinical and ethical scenarios, so can an individual's view of norms (Haslam et al. 2005). Social identification can also lead to norms within a group that make effective teamwork with other groups difficult (Horsburgh et al. 2006). For example, doctors may value working as individuals, while nurses may value work that is more collective (Horsburgh et al. 2006). In this context, health professionals may need to form new interprofessional in-groups in situations such as caring for a difficult patient or managing a busy clinic.

The characteristics of the medical profession are changing with time. For example, being patient-centered and empathic is more valued than it was in the past, and paternalism is less accepted (R. L. Cruess and Cruess 2016b; Irvine 2016). The social identity framework is flexible, and therefore can accommodate the dynamic nature of "what it means to be a doctor." Social identity theory and social complexity theories predict that, given the institutional support for diversity, it may become easier for females and individuals from ethnic minorities to feel that they fit into the in-group. Correspondingly, social identity theory predicts that as learners incorporate the values of the profession, they adopt new values and behaviors that lead them to challenge the status quo (Hafferty et al. 2016).

Follow-Up to the Case of Jessica

During Jessica's fourth year of medical school as she transitioned to internship, she enrolled in an evening mindfulness meditation class at the university. There she met other health professionals and became interested in spirituality. She arranged to shadow Susan, a second-year resident in internal medicine whom she had worked with during her internal medicine clerkship. During her previous experience working with Susan, she was focused on learning about diseases; now, she was able to observe how Susan organized her daily work activities and how she conducted difficult conversations with patients.

Once at her residency program, Jessica felt buoyed by her experience with Susan. She joined the weekly lunchtime intern support group to help her to bond with others (her new in-group). She found a mentor, Angela, an older female colleague who shared her interest in spirituality and health, and introduced her to a meditation group at the hospital. She met with Angela regularly for dinner to reflect on the challenging experiences of her internship.

Later, as Jessica transitioned from resident to attending, she found it harder to build a support group. She had to look outside of her specialty and her institution to find other new attendings like herself. However, she joined a staff committee on wellness, and was able to find a group of female physicians who tackled the difficulties of working as a physician and being a mother. She felt her isolation dissipate over time as she developed a new sense of teamwork with these colleagues. Eventually, Jessica was able to understand how her multiple identities (mom, clinician, teacher, Asian minority, Buddhist) intersected in different ways at different times. Six years later, Jessica has two kids and is now working as an assistant professor. She has a large practice base and is a popular physician with the Chinese and Korean community where she works. She bought a house in a diverse area close to her practice. She joined a nearby Buddhist temple which is active in community service and interfaith activities. While interviewing another young woman candidate for a faculty position at her institution she said:

"I am very happy at this institution. Of course it is never easy juggling motherhood with clinical practice and teaching but my meditation group and my patients keep me going at work and my neighborhood mom's group keeps be going at home."

Final Thoughts: Conceptualizing Theory to Practice

We recognize three ways in which medical educators influence PIF (Crossley and Vivekananda-Schmidt 2009; Gude et al. 2005). The first is through knowledge—explicitly teaching theories of PIF. Some have argued that such teaching is important to improve learners' understanding of their own professional identity development (Sternszus 2016). Learners gain an understanding about the attributes and values of the medical profession and the relationship between the medical profession and society (that is, the social contract). They can use the theoretical frameworks to understand how (and sometimes why) they have reached their current stage of development. This teaching can also anticipate their future professional development. Explicitly examining the concept of individual identity and social identity can help learners work through difficult experiences in their training, such as the identity transitions from student to physician, the role as physicians in a patient-physician dyad, or the transition from doctors-in-training to attending physicians.

The second way to promote PIF is through workplace practice or situated learning. Learners work alongside role models and have a chance to "play the role of physician" before having the skills and knowledge to be a physician or adopting the identity of a physician. Role playing in a real-world clinical environment leads to the development of identity and behaviors of a professional with the experience leading to competence, accompanied by an enhanced sense of self, as well as satisfaction and joy (R. L. Cruess et al. 2015, p. 723).

Thirdly, feedback from patients, role models, and peers helps to shape professional identity (Irvine 2016). Feedback can be about performance in clinical settings or about reflections on critical experiences (S. R. Cruess and Cruess 2016a). We theorize that the feedback can be reassuring to the learner that they are indeed part of the in-group of professionals. This may also provide useful observations to make clear to a learner why the in-group has not yet accepted them as a member.

Questions for Future Research

The evidence base for professional identity development in medical education is just beginning to appear. As Monrouxe (2010) notes, "If we want to know how our curricula impact on the development of tomorrow's doctors we must develop a sensitivity to the ways in which identities are constructed, enacted, invoked, or exploited in a variety of interactional settings," both formal and informal (Monrouxe 2010, p. 45). Research applying social identity theory to nursing education has been more common (Currie et al. 2010; Oaker and Brown 1986).

> One area for future research is studying medical students' narratives about their experiences in training to understand how they develop their professional identities.
>
> Social identity theory can also be used to study how in-groups can be utilized to enhance functioning of teams in medical education with increasing diversity, emphasis on teamwork, and interprofessional education.

References

American Board of Internal Medicine (ABIM) Foundation, American College of Physicians-American Society of Internal Medicine (ACP-ASIM) Foundation; and European Federation of Internal Medicine. (2002). Medical Professionalism in the new millennium: A physician charter. *Annals of Internal Medicine* 136(3): 243–246. doi: 10.7326/0003-4819-136-3-200202050-00012.

Abrams, D. E., and Hogg, M. A. (eds.). (1990). *Social identity theory: Constructive and critical advances.* New York: Springer-Verlag.

Allport, G. W. (1979). *The nature of prejudice: The classic study of the roots of discrimination.* New York: Basic Books.

American Board of Medical Specialties (ABMS) Board of Directors. (2012). *ABMS definition of medical professionalism (long form).* Chicago: American Board of Medical Specialties.

Berzonsky, M. D. (1989). The self as a theorist: Individual differences in identity formation. *International Journal of Personal Construct Psychology* 2(4): 363–376. doi: 10.1080/08936038908404746.

Brewer, M. B. (2001). The many faces of social identity: Implications for political psychology. *Political Psychology* 22(1): 115–125. doi: 10.1111/0162-895x.00229.

Burford, B. (2012). Group processes in medical education: Learning from social identity theory. *Medical Education* 46(2): 143–152. doi: 10.1111/j.1365-2923.2011.04099.x.

Crossley, J., and Vivekananda-Schmidt, P. (2009). The development and evaluation of a Professional Self Identity Questionnaire to measure evolving professional self-identity in health and social care students. *Medical Teacher* 31(12). doi: 10.3109/01421590903193547.

Cruess, S. R., and Cruess, R. L. (2016a). General principles for establishing programs to support professionalism and professional identity formation at the undergraduate and postgraduate levels. In R. L. Cruess, S. R. Cruess, and Y. Steinert (eds.), *Teaching Medical Professionalism,* 2nd ed. (pp. 113–123). Cambridge: Cambridge University Press.

Cruess, R. L., and Cruess, S. R. (2016b). Professionalism and professional identity formation: The cognitive base. In R. L. Cruess, S. R. Cruess, and Y. Steinert (eds.), *Teaching Medical Professionalism,* 2nd ed. (pp. 5–25). Cambridge: Cambridge University Press.

Cruess, R. L., Cruess, S. R., Boudreau, J. D., Snell, L., and Steinert, Y. (2014). Reframing medical education to support professional identity formation. *Academic Medicine* 89(11): 1446–1451. doi: 10.1097/acm.0000000000000427.

Cruess, R. L., Cruess, S. R., Boudreau, J. D., Snell, L., and Steinert, Y. (2015). A schematic representation of the professional identity formation and socialization of medical students and residents. *Academic Medicine* 90(6): 718–725. doi: 10.1097/acm.0000000000000700.

Cruess, R. L., Cruess, S. R., and Steinert, Y. (2016). Amending Miller's pyramid to include professional identity formation. *Academic Medicine* 91(2): 180–185. doi: 10.1097/acm.0000000000000913.

Currie, G., Finn, R., and Martin, G. (2010). Role transition and the interaction of relational and social identity: New nursing roles in the English NHS. *Organization Studies* 31(7): 941–961. doi: 10.1177/0170840610373199.

Erikson, E. H. (1994). *Identity: Youth and crisis.* New York: NY: Norton.

Gjerberg, E., and Kjølsrød, L. (2001). The doctor-nurse relationship: How easy is it to be a female doctor co-operating with a female nurse? *Social Science and Medicine* 52(2): 189–202. doi: 10.1016/s0277-9536(00)00219-7.

Goldie, J. (2012). The formation of professional identity in medical students: Considerations for educators. *Medical Teacher* 34(9): e641-e648. doi: 10.3109/0142159x.2012.687476.

Gude, T., Vaglum, P., Tyssen, R., Ekeberg, Ø., Hem, E., Røvik, J. O., . . . Grønvold, N. T. (2005). Identification with the role of doctor at the end of medical school: A nationwide longitudinal study. *Medical Education* 39(1): 66–74. doi: 10.1111/j.1365–2929.2004.02034.x.

Hafferty, F. W., Michalec, B., Martimianakis, M. A., and Tilburt, J. C. (2016). Alternative framings, countervailing visions: Locating the "p" in professional identity formation. *Academic Medicine* 91(2): 171–174. doi: 10.1097/acm.0000000000000961.

Harvill, L. M. (1981). Anticipatory socialization of medical students. *Academic Medicine* 56(5): 431–433. doi: 10.1097/00001888-198105000-00009.

Haslam, S. A., O'Brien, A., Jetten, J., Vormedal, K., and Penna, S. (2005). Taking the strain: Social identity, social support, and the experience of stress. *British Journal of Social Psychology* 44(3): 355–370. doi: 10.1348/014466605 × 37468.

Helmich, E., and Dornan, T. (2012). Do you really want to be a doctor? The highs and lows of identity development. *Medical Education* 46(2): 132–134. doi: 10.1111/j.1365–2923.2011.04189.x.

Hogg, M. A., and Reid, S. A. (2006). Social identity, self-categorization, and the communication of group norms. *Communication Theory* 16(1): 7–30. doi: 10.1111/j.1468–2885.2006.00003.x.

Hornsey, M. J. (2008). Social identity theory and self-categorization theory: A historical review. *Social and Personality Psychology Compass* 2(1): 204–222. doi: 10.1111/j.1751–9004.2007.00066.x.

Horsburgh, M., Perkins, R., Coyle, B., and Degeling, P. (2006). The professional subcultures of students entering medicine, nursing and pharmacy programmes. *Journal of Interprofessional Care* 20(4): 425–431. doi: 10.1080/13561820600805233.

Irby, D. M., and Hamstra, S. J. (2016). Parting the clouds: Three professionalism frameworks in medical education. *Academic Medicine* 91(12): 1606–1611. doi: 10.1097/acm.0000000000001190.

Irvine, S. D. (2016). Professionalism, professional identity, and licensing and accrediting bodies. In R. L. Cruess, S. R. Cruess, and Y. Steinert (eds.), *Teaching medical professionalism,* 2nd ed. (pp. 201–216). Cambridge: Cambridge University Press.

Jarvis-Selinger, S., Pratt, D. D., and Regehr, G. (2012). Competency is not enough: Integrating identity formation into the medical education discourse. *Academic Medicine,* 87(9): 1185–1190. doi: 10.1097/acm.0b013e3182604968.

Kegan, R. (1982). *The evolving self: Problem and process in human development.* Cambridge, MA: Harvard University Press.

Kirk, L. M. (2007). Professionalism in medicine: Definitions and considerations for teaching. *Baylor University Medical Center Proceedings* 20(1) 13–16.

Kumagai, A. K. (2010). Commentary: Forks in the road: Disruption and transformation in professional development. *Academic Medicine* 85(12): 1819–1820. doi: 10.1097/acm.0b013e3181fa2a59.

Lloyd, J. V., Schneider, J., Scales, K., Bailey, S., and Jones, R. (2011). Ingroup identity as an obstacle to effective multiprofessional and interprofessional teamwork: Findings from an ethnographic study of healthcare assistants in dementia care. *Journal of Interprofessional Care* 25(5): 345–351. doi: 10.3109/13561820.2011.567381.

Marcia, J. E. (1993). The ego identity status approach to ego identity. *Ego Identity* 3–21. doi: 10.1007/978-1-4613-8330-7_1.

Miles-Johnson, T. (2015). Policing diversity: Examining police resistance to training reforms for transgender people in Australia. *Journal of Homosexuality* 63(1): 103–136. doi: 10.1080/00918369.2015.1078627.

Monrouxe, L. V. (2009). Negotiating professional identities: Dominant and contesting narratives in medical students' longitudinal audio diaries. *Current Narratives* 1(1): 41–59.

Monrouxe, L. V. (2010). Identity, identification and medical education: Why should we care? *Medical Education* 44(1): 40–49. doi: 10.1111/j.1365-2923.2009.03440.x.

Monrouxe, L. V. (2015). When I say . . . intersectionality in medical education research. *Medical Education* 49(1): 21–22. doi: 10.1111/medu.12428.

Monrouxe, L. V. (2016). Theoretical insights into the nature and nurture of professional identities. In R. L. Cruess, S. R. Cruess, and Y. Steinert (eds.), *Teaching medical professionalism,* 2nd ed. (pp. 37–53). Cambridge: Cambridge University Press.

Monrouxe, L., and Rees, C. E. (2017). *Healthcare professionalism: Improving practice through reflections on workplace dilemmas.* Oxford: Wiley-Blackwell.

Monrouxe, L. V., Rees, C. E., and Hu, W. (2011). Differences in medical students' explicit discourses of professionalism: Acting, representing, becoming. *Medical Education* 45(6): 585–602. doi: 10.1111/j.1365-2923.2010.03878.x.

Oaker, G., and Brown, R. (1986). Intergroup relations in a hospital setting: A further test of social identity theory. *Human Relations* 39(8): 767–778. doi: 10.1177/001872678603900804.

Rees, C. E., and Knight, L. V. (2007). Viewpoint: The trouble with assessing students' professionalism: Theoretical insights from sociocognitive psychology. *Academic Medicine* 82(1): 46–50. doi: 10.1097/01.acm.0000249931.85609.05.

Roccas, S., and Brewer, M. B. (2002). Social identity complexity. *Personality and Social Psychology Review* 6(2): 88–106. doi: 10.1207/s15327957pspr0602_01.

Savelkoul, M., Hewstone, M., Scheepers, P., and Stolle, D. (2015). Does relative out-group size in neighborhoods drive down associational life of Whites in the U.S.? Testing constrict, conflict and contact theories. *Social Science Research* 52, 236–252. doi: 10.1016/j.ssresearch.2015.01.013.

Schaik, S. M., O'Sullivan, P. S., Eva, K. W., Irby, D. M., and Regehr, G. (2016). Does source matter? Nurses' and physicians' perceptions of interprofessional feedback. *Medical Education* 50(2): 181–188. doi: 10.1111/medu.12850.

Sternszus, R. (2016). Developing a professional identity: A learner's perspective. In R. L. Cruess, S. R. Cruess, and Y. Steinert (eds.), *Teaching Medical Professionalism*, 2nd ed. (pp. 26–36). Cambridge: Cambridge University Press.

Tajfel, H. (2010). *Social identity and intergroup relations*. Cambridge: Cambridge University Press.

Tsouroufli, M., Rees, C. E., Monrouxe, L. V., and Sundaram, V. (2011). Gender, identities and intersectionality in medical education research. *Medical Education* 45(3): 213–216. doi: 10.1111/j.1365-2923.2010.03908.x.

Turner, J. C., Oakes, P. J., Haslam, S. A., and McGarty, C. (1994). Self and collective: Cognition and social context. In T. Postmes and N. R. Branscombe (eds.), *Rediscovering social identity: Key readings* (pp. 287–299). New York: Psychology Press.

Westerman, M., Teunissen, P. W., van der Vleuten, C. P., Scherpbier, A. J., Siegert, C. E., van der Lee, N. V., and Scheele, F. (2010). Understanding the transition from resident to attending physician: A transdisciplinary, qualitative study. *Academic Medicine* 85(12): 1914–1919. doi: 10.1097/acm.0b013e3181fa2913.

Wilson, I., Cowin, L. S., Johnson, M., and Young, H. (2013). Professional identity in medical students: Pedagogical challenges to medical education. *Teaching and Learning in Medicine* 25(4): 369–373. doi: 10.1080/10401334.2013.827968.

5

Graceful Self-Promotion

An Approach for Career Development

KATHERINE N. HUBER, ZAREEN ZAIDI, AND PAGE S. MORAHAN[1]

Ad altiora tendo—I strive toward higher things.
Source unknown

In this chapter we describe the self-promotion as a strategy for academic advancement and to ensure individual visibility in an institution. Barriers to self-promotion in particular cultural and gender issues are described and readers will find clear strategies to practice self-promotion.

Objectives

Identify barriers that potentially hinder career advancement.
Develop strategies to practice graceful self-promotion.
Use these skills to help mentor colleagues and trainees.

Heena is a 38-year-old pediatrician who practices in a large academic tertiary-care system. She completed medical school in Nepal and, after completing USMLE steps with commendable scores, she joined a prestigious teaching program in New York City. Posttraining, she moved to an academic center in the southern region of the United States, where she soon established a reputation as a stellar worker and excellent clinician. After a few years, Heena was appointed as the director of one of the outpatient clinic sites, overseeing 15 faculty, nursing, and administrative staff.

Heena has had difficulty ensuring that the clinic's administrative rules

1 Katherine N. Huber, M.D., University of Florida College of Medicine, Gainesville, FL.
Zareen Zaidi, M.D., Ph.D., University of Florida College of Medicine, Gainesville, FL.
Page S. Morahan, Ph.D., Drexel University College of Medicine, Philadelphia, PA.

were followed by all clinic faculty members. She worries about how she will be perceived by faculty who have been at the academic center "forever"; that is, some had completed their medical school and residency training there and had later gone on to be faculty. She perceived herself to be an "outsider" and went into staff meetings viewing the "room to be full of white people" and thinking "who was she to tell them what to do?" On occasion, she knew that she should tell a faculty member that their behavior with another staff member was inappropriate and would not be tolerated in the future, but did not do so because she worried about backlash or an outright confrontation. Over the next few years, she remained silent during staff meetings, not volunteering an opinion or managing to project the good work done at her clinic site.

It is not surprising that self-promotion can be challenging for physicians who are looking to advance their career. While they want to make known their successes in the workplace, they are afraid of coming off as aggressive and turning off the people that they are hoping to impress with their accomplishments. Presenting achievements and positive attributes with humility, at appropriate times and situations, can help with career advancement. On the other hand, exaggeration, excessive reminders about accomplishments, and overexuberance can have the opposite effect, especially for women and minorities within an organization (Rudman 1998). Several studies have shown that aggressive self-promoters tend to overestimate the positive effect of their efforts on the person receiving it and underestimate the negative effects (Scopelliti et al.2015). Thus, while it is important for faculty to ensure that their accomplishments receive appropriate recognition, they must deliver the message in a way that colleagues and superiors will not perceive as annoying, aggressive, or bragging. This dilemma led to one of the authors (PSM) to coin the term "graceful self-promotion" (Morahan 2004), a method of making one's accomplishments and abilities visible with tact and humility.

There are two reasons that learning graceful self-promotion is important. First, women and faculty from certain cultures are particularly apt to struggle with self-promotion due to longstanding gender and cultural roles and norms. Second, faculty in general often focus their efforts on excellent performance in their particular microcosm and believe that this alone (without making their accomplishments explicitly public) will give them opportunities for advancement within their departments and medical school. They are then frustrated when they are passed over for leadership positions and other career-advancing positions.

A well-thought-out strategy for graceful self-promotion can be essential for career development. In section 1 of this chapter, we provide insights into cultures that lead to unconscious learning, which hinders self-promotion and can lead to the proverbial "glass ceiling" (Morahan et al. 2011) and the "bamboo ceiling" (Hewlett et al. 2011; Hyun 2012). In section 2, we provide tips for faculty to practice graceful self-promotion.

Understanding Cultural and Gender Conflicts

Graceful self-promotion in dependent and interdependent cultures

Culture plays a significant role in how physicians view themselves and their role in the workplace. Markus and Conner (Markus and Conner 2014) assert that all people have an inner "self" or sense of being, which controls how an individual acts and reacts to the world around them. Since different cultures promote different views of how individuals should behave and interact with society, an individual's upbringing strongly influences this inner "self." This influence is evident in the cultural differences between East and West, as well as gender, racial/ethnic, and socioeconomic class differences, to name a few. As a general rule, Eastern, African and Latino cultures, women, and the lower socioeconomic class tend to uphold an interdependent value system. In such interdependent cultures, people tend to be raised to feel that their relationships with others are of primary importance; they tend to be rooted in tradition, obligation, and concern about the effect of their actions on others (Markus and Kitayama 1991). In contrast, the independent culture value system typical of Western and white cultures, men, and the upper socioeconomic class encourages individualism, uniqueness, and self-confidence, and focuses less on the impact that an individual's decisions have on those around them (Table 3) (Markus and Conner 2014).

Although both independent and interdependent cultures are equally thoughtful, emotional and active, differences in opinion and conflicts can arise because of the subtle differences in thoughts, feelings, and actions of individuals in response to the same situation. As a faculty mentor, it is important to first appreciate the complexity of one's own "self"; this involves training one's self to: avoid default assumptions about people on the other side of the cultural divide; ask questions; judge more slowly; and act more carefully and intentionally. Strategies or techniques to improve relationships and therefore performance when dealing with interdependent and independent cultures include understanding that interdependent cultures encourage solving problems in silence; therefore if a participant is quiet, it does not indicate that they are "checked-out." In contrast, participants from independent cultures may prefer to solve a problem while speaking.

In general, interdependent cultures encourage leveraging harmonious relationships (in family, classrooms, workplace, and society), while independent cultures encourage focusing on one's sense of control. This demonstrates the need to capitalize on both independent and interdependent behaviors, endeavoring to better leverage each other's strengths. Table 4 summarizes strategies that faculty can undertake. For example, interdependents can aspire to speak up more, understanding that they have as much authority as anyone else, and can also develop the mentoring and mentee skills that are typical in the Western setting. Similarly, independents can increase focus on relationship building before jumping into problem solving, learn about other cultures, and work toward a growth mind-set.

Graceful self-promotion and women

While women fall into the interdependent culture group, situational factors unique to each individual make generalization about the career advancement of women difficult. Literature over the past four decades, however, clearly demonstrates that women academics in health professions face more difficulties in career advancement than men, even women medical school deans (Bickel et al. 2002; White et al. 2012). Although women have reached parity at professional entry in many fields, women faculty progress more slowly through academic ranks, and there is persistent gender inequity in leadership (Bickel et al. 2002; Martinez et al. 2007; Nelson and Rogers 2003; Wright et al. 2003). Near parity at entry for the past two decades has not had the expected positive impact on advancement to senior leadership, demonstrating that the pipeline model

(Bickel et al. 2002) is a myth; the proportion of women leaders remains below the critical mass needed for sustainable equity (Morahan et al. 2011; Nelson and Rogers 2003). The paucity of women leaders in turn affects how academic medicine meets the requirements of the growing number of students, faculty, staff, and patients from diverse backgrounds.

Two general issues pertaining to self-promotion contribute to the persistent gender inequity (Morahan et al. 2011). The first encompasses the internal psychological and cultural tenets of women. The second involves institutional policies and procedures and the sociocultural norms that contain individuals, families, academic health institutions within the United States.

Women faculty need to address the internal messages that impede effective graceful self-promotion. Labelled a variety of ways—"advancement reticence" (Ross-Smith and Chesterman 2009), low self-efficacy (Sloma-Williams et al. 2009), Girl Syndrome (Ross-Smith and Chesterman 2009), self-imposed glass ceiling (Austin 2009), Imposter Syndrome, Tiara Syndrome (Fitzpatrick and Curran 2014), and role identity incongruity (Fletcher 2001)—all diminish women's effectiveness, as well as that of minority groups, in the male-dominated academic medicine world (Davidhizar and Lonser 2004; Ely and Meyerson 2000; Fitzpatrick and Curran 2014; Fletcher 2001). Women tend not to pursue promotional opportunities for various reasons, including a lack of self-confidence to apply without encouragement from others, particularly those in positions of leadership (Morahan et al. 2011; Odom et al. 2007). They may focus on all of their perceived weaknesses and not share their accomplishments (Davidhizar and Lonser 2004; Odom et al. 2007). Inhibitory internal messages also include cultural family commitment norms and perceived incongruity between dual identity as a woman and a leader.

The Tiara Syndrome is the tendency in women (and also many men and minorities) to focus solely on job performance, believing this is sufficient for recognition and promotion (Fitzpatrick and Curran 2014). Instead of self-promotion and active pursuit of opportunities, they wait to be recognized, and for opportunities to come to them (to be presented with the "tiara"). They are often bypassed for opportunities because they have not made themselves and their accomplishments visible to those around them.

Addressing these internal issues, however, is not sufficient, because women faculty (and minorities) work within institutional policies and procedures, and all are embedded in both the traditional academic health center culture and sociocultural norms (Babaria et al. 2012; Magrane et al. 2012). A comprehensive approach that combines Ely and Myerson's (2000) framework with the leadership continuum (Morahan et al. 2011) provides a neutral process for addressing gender equity.

The first of the framework's four approaches equips women through professional development, strategic career planning, and mentoring initiatives to address skill deficiencies and self-confidence. Despite excellent credentials, women tend to lack the skills to showcase their abilities and actively pursue opportunities at the next level.

The second approach is creating equal opportunities; examples include a formal funded women's advancement office, an annual published report card on the status of women, and policies and procedures to address barriers in advancement that disproportionately affect women, such as childbirth, adoption, and parental responsibilities.

The third approach is increasing the visibility of women's accomplishments and valuation of women's skills. This approach requires action at both at the institutional level as well as with individual women, developing skills to increase their visibility, be successful mentees and mentors, and build collaborative networks with other faculty and leaders.

The fourth approach is the most challenging to address—institutional culture change for sustained gender equity. This approach involves commitment of highly visible leaders (leader champions) with strategic plans and accountability for building a gender-inclusive institution (Ely and Meyerson 2000).

Tips for Graceful Self-Promotion

Tip 1: Develop a mind-set of generativity

Health professions educators often focus passionately on clinical work and are very successful in their respective fields but they lack visibility at an institutional, local, or national level. Faculty at academic centers often misperceive self-promotion as a form of bragging or arrogance (Berman et al. 2015; Scopelliti et al. 2015). However, research about prosocial behavior and generosity shows that bragging about personal achievements does not affect how others perceive an individual's intrinsic motivation (Berman et al. 2015). Furthermore, those who self-promote have greater career satisfaction than those who do not (Cheng et al. 2014). In a recent study, deans of U.S medical schools noted that the most common characteristic differentiating "Rock Stars in Academic Medicine" from other faculty was the ability to self-promote (Lucey et al. 2010).

Learning the art of graceful self-promotion is essential at the clinical, academic, administrative, and society levels (Bleier and Kann 2013). This skill requires you to view self-promotion through a different lens—that of generativity (Komives et al. 2006), the ability to look beyond oneself and express commitment for the welfare of others (Ho and Odom 2015; Lieff 2010). This reframing can be a useful lens for educators regarding self-promotion. When self-promoting, you are:

Educating/engaging others—NOT selling to them

Helping your organization or department look good through your success

Positively impacting the larger group by being generous with praise and gratitude to others

Role-modeling and mentoring others in the skill of graceful self-promotion

Tip 2: Consider graceful self-promotion as part of your strategic career management

Goal setting

Given the challenges faculty face in advancing their careers, especially the heavy clinical, research, or educational workloads, it is important to have a plan to attain short-, medium-, and long-term goals (Bleier and Kann 2013; Clark 2012). Just as politicians have a long-term campaign strategy to attain their career goals—reaching out to supporters, building and exercising influence, and then executing relentlessly—faculty can devise their own long-term plan for their career paths (Clark 2012). The first step is to set clear goals—personal, clinical, research, and educational—with clear timelines (that is, short-, medium-, and long-term) (Bleier and Kann 2013). The next step is to strategize the how, when, and where self-promotion could be achieved—gracefully!

Networks

The importance of networks is three-fold: they serve as support groups, they can be a mentoring system, and they can be useful for strategic partnerships that amplify individual accomplishments. Social support groups, as well as formal and informal mentoring relationships, have been shown to be important for academic success of students and faculty, particularly for minority groups (Buddeberg-Fischer and Herta 2006; Dobkin and Hutchinson 2013; Zea et al. 1995). Morzinski and Fisher (2002) reported that successful primary care faculty initiated on the average nine mentoring relationships with colleagues—typically three peers, two mentors, one academic consultant, and three additional colleagues perceived available for future support.

As in the business world (Clark 2012), making a Power Map (Figure 4) can help you proactively identify your support group. The process can identify people who can have an impact on your career, then enable you to intentionally develop or nurture relationships with those most influential in helping you meet and work with key contacts. Very importantly, you can use network contacts as strategic third parties who can present the desirable information on your behalf (Pfeffer et al. 2006).

You may need to supply a list of colleagues when you are up for academic promotion. Use the following tips to become known by over 10 external people. You can use the communications you prepare (see Tip 3) when you interact with these individuals.

At meetings, look over the agenda, and target individuals to meet.

Proactively plan breakfasts, coffee, or teatime with the key people you want to connect with.

Always wear your name tag at meetings and reintroduce yourself.

When interacting with these people, establish rapport. This might include: commenting on an article of theirs, referring to people they know, and following up by sending relevant works of your own.

On campus, meet visiting speakers and drive them to and from the airport, hotel, and campus.

Be active on listservs and other electronic media used in your disciplinary groups.

Join and be active in subcommittees of disciplinary societies.

In summary, for successful graceful self-promotion as part of a strategic career plan:

Be sensitive to timing, place, and people involved.

Don't wait until the annual review; rather, keep your boss and other major stakeholders in the loop.

Regularly forward your accomplishments (for example, publications, invitations, teaching evaluations) to your chair with a note. The rationale in the note might be: "I thought that this might look good for department annual report," or "Just wanted you to see this. You must be proud of what you have helped start in education."

In the spirit of generativity, send your boss or others higher up notes of thanks or congratulations for their accomplishments. It's amazing how little recognition one gets from one's direct reports; they will notice!

Remember, self-promotion will help prevent credit theft.

Reinforcing from Tip 1, build your social networks and partnerships, so that you can strategically use third-person parties to promote each other's accomplishments. You can also nominate colleagues (and students) for awards. Make sure friendly peers know you and promote you (you do the same). The goal is to promote each other.

Make sure that key people know what you've done lately and how it helps THEM or the unit.

Be visible (for example, get on the "radar screen" of people you want to develop relationships with).

Tip 3: Become a skilled and strategic communicator to gracefully self-promote and increase your visibility

The tips below come from the experience of the last author in teaching in leadership programs over the last two decades. We thank participants of a workshop at the Association of American Medical Colleges' Early Women in Medicine Professional Development Seminar, December 2005, for a number of these tips.

First, develop several kinds of oral communications. In all of these, remember: Stories Sell while Facts Tell (Morahan 2004). So, whenever speaking (see types below), include a very brief story that engages your audience!

Develop a succinct story (5–7-minute maximum), using the STAR format: S = situation/challenge/opportunity; TA= task: what you or your team did; and R = results.

Be ready also for very brief (30-second to 2-minute) hallway and "elevator" versions of your STAR. They are quick speeches conveying what you are working on, achievements, and support needed.

Take risks to present at seminars, lectures, and grand rounds. While these are longer communications, it's still useful to use stories and the STAR strategy—as you describe something that your research team has accomplished, for example.

Another issue is how to make your communications more visible. In strategizing about this:

Don't be stingy with your information. Remember that it might give others ideas for collaboration with you, or serve as a model to encourage others to tell their accomplishments.

Report your accomplishments in a variety of media (for example, institutional newsletter, department website, personal professional website).

Start a publication board in the hall. Display local posters in a highly trafficked area. Post pertinent articles from the local newsletter or internal publication on the departmental bulletin board. This is in addition Tip 1, sending this type of accomplishment via snail mail or email to your bosses, colleagues, and other people interested in your career.

Become skilled with the electronic media communication tools that are common in your school and discipline (for example, webinars, videoconferencing, websites, listservs, blogs, Wikis, Dropbox, Instagram, LinkedIn, and so on).

Tip 4: Consider your personal style—how to be "comfortable in your skin"—how to "be an authentic powerful person"

Authentic individuals learn from life experiences and practice their values consistently. They are the same person in all aspects of life—personal, work, community (George et al. 2007). The following steps may help:

Recognize, leverage, and flex your introversion (Cain 2013) or extraversion. For introverts, this means becoming comfortable with being a "situational extrovert" since this is the norm in U.S. society. Tips include: be rested before you go to large group events, prepare your key self-promotion points and communication, and have a few people in mind to focus on conversing with. With your communication at the ready, you can gracefully self-promote!

Develop an authentic powerful style that may include "dressing for success."

Prepare yourself emotionally, so you remain calm (for example, perhaps find someone safe, outside of work, to whom you can vent to; develop a meditation practice or reflective practice to process life events, or develop a physical movement practice).

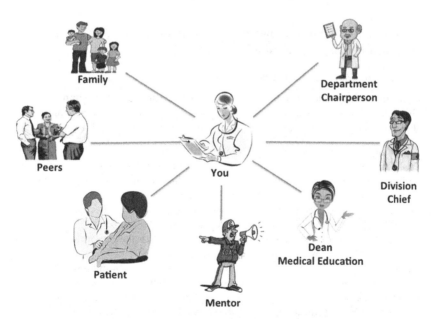

Figure 4. Power map of your career campaign. Adapted from D. Clark, A campaign strategy for your career, *Harvard Business Review* 90, no. 11: 131–134, 151.

In conclusion, strategically planning and being sensitive to timing (Morahan 2004), place, and people can produce a successful combination of graceful self-promotion and humility (Giacalone and Rosenfeld 1986; Scopelliti et al. 2015).

Table 3. Cultural conflicts

Independent Cultures	Interdependent Cultures
CHARACTERISTICS	
• Individual	• Relational
• Unique	• Similar
• Influencing	• Adjusting
• Free	• Rooted
• Equal (yet great!)	• Ranked
RELATIONAL CHARACTERISTICS	
• Solid edges	• Porous edges
• Separate circles of self and others	• Intersecting circles of self and others
• Focus on one's self	(relational, rooted, ranked)
	• Focus on one's relationships

Adapted from Markus and Conner (2014).

Table 4. Strategies for teaching/learning and leading/managing with interdependent and independent cultures

Strategies for Teaching/Learning and Leading/Managing

How can interdependent people plug into independence to be better able to collaborate in the world?	How can independent people tap into the power of interdependence to prepare for a more competitive marketplace?
• Speak up.	• Listen.
• Ask for help.	• Think about how you are similar to others.
• Think about how you are different from others.	• Remember that adjusting to others does not mean you're weak.
• Remember that asserting yourself doesn't mean you're selfish.	• Consider how each action affects others.
• Consider each action as a choice.	• Ask people what they need.
• Assume you have as much authority as others.	• Partner with local institutions instead of imposing your own.
• Reward competence.	• Place relationships first, business second.
• Look for options.	• Accurately portray the other in the media.
• Get mentoring and education for leadership skills in independent societies.	• Go outside comfort zone to experience interdependent cultures.
	• Assume that others have more authority than you.

- Visualize a "possible self" into reality: plot timelines, likely setbacks, strategies to overcome them including leveraging interdependent relationships with families and communities.
- Ask successful interdependents to describe how their interdependent ways (e.g., fear of asking questions in public) initially caused them difficulties, and what independent strategies worked (e.g., speaking in public, asking for help).

- Rather than use Socratic *cold-call* methods, *warm-call*: alert participants ahead of time that you will call on them to share their ideas, or convene in small groups to foster sharing.
- Use the jigsaw model to foster interdependent skills: split the group into diverse groups of 6–8; assign each member one of 6–8 units to study independently; form back to diverse group where each member shares; hold group accountable for learning or performance.
- Align materials (readings, videos, letters, etc.) that reflect the diversity in the group.
- Reframe usual approaches: Discuss vs. argue; raise a challenge vs. throw down a competition; go for the gold vs. go for the jugular; and we vs. I.
- Value people equally with results: spend time necessary to make/maintain relationships; pay attention to own/others' relational styles/social needs.
- Educate the whole student with offerings of science, music, and art.
- Develop *grit* in learners by adding Eastern growth mind-set approach to Western fixed mind-set approach about talent and intelligence; praise students for effort, help develop realistic account of failures, and work to meet high standards.
- Work harder to accommodate work styles of those from interdependent cultures; to contribute ideas in writing or informal sessions, in order to shine without undue stress.
- Realize that time spent on defending oneself against threats is time not spent on more productive pursuits.

Adapted from Markus and Conner (2014).

Final Thoughts and Conceptual Framework

Our conceptual framework for this chapter derives from long experience in academic leadership development, strategic career planning, and academic faculty affairs (PSM), together with the robust literature on strategic career management and communication skills (Chambers 1999; Ibarra et al. 2010), and the impact of diversity in learning and career advancement (Sue et al. 2007). Figure 5 describes two key steps in graceful self-promotion.

Step 1: Understand yourself and reflect on cultural upbringing, since different cultures promote different views of how individuals should behave and interact with society. We then suggest using Table 4 to explore strategies for Teaching/Learning and Leading/Managing with Interdependent and Independent Cultures.

Step 2: Strategically use the tips for graceful self-promotion described in detail in section 2.

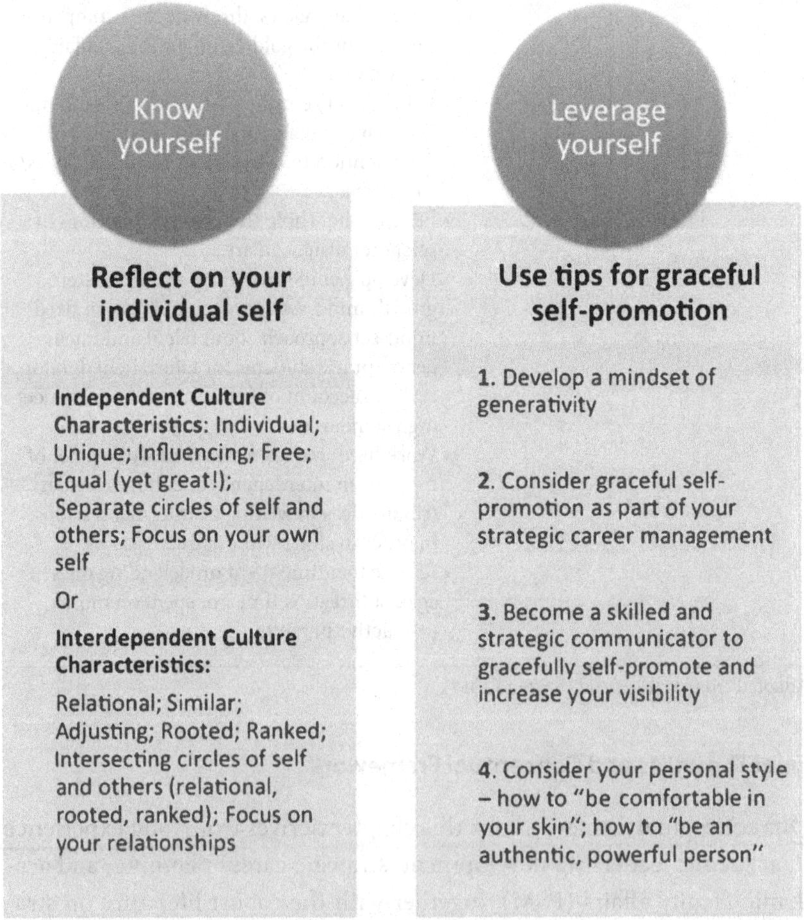

Know yourself

Leverage yourself

Reflect on your individual self

Independent Culture Characteristics: Individual; Unique; Influencing; Free; Equal (yet great!); Separate circles of self and others; Focus on your own self

Or

Interdependent Culture Characteristics:

Relational; Similar; Adjusting; Rooted; Ranked; Intersecting circles of self and others (relational, rooted, ranked); Focus on your relationships

Use tips for graceful self-promotion

1. Develop a mindset of generativity

2. Consider graceful self-promotion as part of your strategic career management

3. Become a skilled and strategic communicator to gracefully self-promote and increase your visibility

4. Consider your personal style – how to "be comfortable in your skin"; how to "be an authentic, powerful person"

Figure 5. Conceptual framework for graceful self-promotion. Figure by authors.

Questions for Future Research

Two areas appear to be fertile ground for faculty development regarding graceful self-promotion:

First, the faculty support groups and mentorship programs that exist in most medical schools could implement the strategies outlined in this chapter to help faculty become aware of the importance of graceful self-promotion and develop the necessary skills.

Second, schools could establish faculty development programs specifically aimed at faculty from Eastern cultures (or other interdependent culture groups) to assist in their development in Western medical schools. With either of these faculty development approaches, researchers will need to conduct longitudinal evaluation research studies to identify the impact of these programs on the advancement of faculty (Dannels et al. 2008; McDade et al. 2004).

References

Austin, L. (2009). *What's holding you back?: 8 critical choices for women's success.* New York, NY: Basic Books.

Babaria, P., Abedin, S., Berg, D., and Nunez-Smith, M. (2012). "I'm too used to it": A longitudinal qualitative study of third year female medical students' experiences of gendered encounters in medical education. *Social Science & Medicine* 74(7): 1013–1020. doi: 10.1016/j.socscimed.2011.11.043.

Berman, J. Z., Levine, E. E., Barasch, A., and Small, D. A. (2015). The Braggart's dilemma: On the social rewards and penalties of advertising prosocial behavior. *Journal of Marketing Research* 52(1): 90–104. doi: 10.1509/jmr.14.0002.

Bickel, J., Wara, D., Atkinson, B. F., Cohen, L. S., Dunn, M., Hostler, S., et al. (2002). Increasing women's leadership in academic medicine: Report of the AAMC project implementation committee. *Academic Medicine* 77(10): 1043–1061.

Bleier, J., and Kann, B. (2013). Academic goals in surgery. *Clinics in Colon and Rectal Surgery* 26(04): 212–217. doi: 10.1055/s-0033-1356719.

Buddeberg-Fischer, B., and Herta, K. (2006). Formal mentoring programmes for medical students and doctors—A review of the Medline literature. *Medical Teacher* 28(3): 248–257. doi: 10.1080/01421590500313043.

Cain, S. (2013). *Quiet: The power of introverts in a world that can't stop talking.* New York, NY: Broadway Books.

Chambers, H. (1999). *Getting promoted: Real strategies for advancing your career.* Reading, MA: Perseus Books.

Cheng, J., Chiu, W., Chang, Y., and Johnstone, S. (2014). Do you put your best foot forward? Interactive effects of task performance and impression management tactics on career outcomes. *Journal of Psychology* 148(6): 621–640. doi: 10.1080/00223980.2013.818929.

Clark, D. (2012). A campaign strategy for your career. *Harvard Business Review* 90(11): 131–134, 151.

Dannels, S. A., Yamagata, H., Mcdade, S. A., Chuang, Y., Gleason, K. A., Mclaughlin, J. M., et al. (2008). Evaluating a leadership program: A comparative, longitudinal study to assess the impact of the Executive Leadership in Academic Medicine (ELAM) program for women. *Academic Medicine* 83(5): 488–495. doi: 10.1097/acm.0b013e31816be551.

Davidhizar, R., and Lonser, G. Y. (2004). Self-promotion: A strategy for career advancement. *Health Care Manager* 23(1): 11–14.

Dobkin, P. L., and Hutchinson, T. A. (2013). Teaching mindfulness in medical school: Where are we now and where are we going? *Medical Education* 47(8): 768–779. doi: 10.1111/medu.12200.

Ely, R. J., and Meyerson, D. E. (2000). Advancing gender equity in organizations: The challenge and importance of maintaining a gender narrative. *Organization* 7(4): 589–608. doi: 10.1177/135050840074005.

Fitzpatrick, T. A., and Curran, C. R. (2014). Waiting for your coronation: A career-limiting trap. *Nursing Economics* 32(3): 162.

Fletcher, J. K. (2001). *Disappearing acts: Gender, power and relational practice at work.* Cambridge, MA: MIT Press.

George, B., Sims, P., McLean, A. N., and Mayer, D. (2007). Discovering your authentic leadership. *Harvard Business Review* 85(2): 129–130, 132–138, 157.

Giacalone, R. A., and Rosenfeld, P. (1986). Self-presentation and self-promotion in an organizational setting. *Journal of Social Psychology* 126(3): 321–326. doi: 10.1080/00224545.1986.9713592.

Hewlett, S., Rashid, R., Forster, D., and Ho, C. (2011). *Asians in America: Unleashing the potential of the "model minority."* New York: Center for Work-Life Policy.

Ho, S. P., and Odom, S. F. (2015). Mindsets of leadership education undergraduates: An approach to program assessment. *Journal of Leadership Education* 13(3). doi: 10.12806/v14/i1/r6.

Hyun, J. (2012). Leadership principles for capitalizing on culturally diverse teams: The bamboo ceiling revisited. *Leader to Leader* 2012(64): 14–19. doi: 10.1002/ltl.20017.

Ibarra, H., Snook, S., and Ramo, L. (2010). Identity-based leader development. In N. Nohria and R. Khurana (eds.), *Handbook of leadership theory and practice* (pp. 657–678). Brighton, MA: Harvard Business Press.

Komives, S. R., Longerbeam, S. D., Owen, J. E., Mainella, F. C., and Osteen, L. (2006). A leadership identity development model: Applications from a grounded theory. *Journal of College Student Development* 47(4): 401–418. doi: 10.1353/csd.2006.0048.

Lieff, S. J. (2010). Faculty development: Yesterday, today and tomorrow: Guide supplement 33.2—Viewpoint. *Medical Teacher* 32(5): 429–431. doi: 10.3109/01421591003677905.

Lucey, C. R., Sedmak, D., Notestine, M., and Souba, W. (2010). Rock stars in academic medicine. *Academic Medicine* 85(8): 1269–1275. doi: 10.1097/acm.0b013e3181e5c0bb.

Magrane, D., Helitzer, D., Morahan, P., Chang, S., Gleason, K., Cardinali, G., and Wu, C. (2012). Systems of career influences: A conceptual model for evaluating the professional development of women in academic medicine. *Journal of Women's Health* 21(12): 1244–1251. doi: 10.1089/jwh.2012.3638.

Markus, H. R., and Conner, A. (2014). *Clash!: How to thrive in a multicultural world.* London: Penguin.

Markus, H. R., and Kitayama, S. (1991). Culture and the self: Implications for cognition, emotion, and motivation. *Psychological Review* 98(2): 224–253. doi: 10.1037//0033-295x.98.2.224.

Martinez, E. D., Botos, J., Dohoney, K. M., Geiman, T. M., Kolla, S. S., Olivera, A., et al. (2007). Falling off the academic bandwagon. Women are more likely to quit at the postdoc to principal investigator transition. *EMBO Reports* 8(11): 977–981. doi: 10.1038/sj.embor.7401110.

McDade, S. A., Richman, R. C., Jackson, G. B., and Morahan, P. S. (2004). Effects of participation in the Executive Leadership in Academic Medicine (ELAM) program on women faculty's perceived leadership capabilities. *Academic Medicine* 79(4): 302–309. doi: 10.1097/00001888-200404000-00005.

Morahan, P. (2004). Graceful self-promotion—It's essential. *Academic Physician and Scientist* 2(3). Retrieved September 12, 2016, from http://www.drexel.edu/medicine/Academics/Womens-Health-and-Leadership/ELAM/Research/ELAM-Publications/#Career.

Morahan, P. S., Rosen, S. E., Richman, R. C., and Gleason, K. A. (2011). The Leadership continuum: A framework for organizational and individual assessment relative to the advancement of women physicians and scientists. *Journal of Women's Health* 20(3): 387–396. doi: 10.1089/jwh.2010.2055.

Morzinski, J. A., and Fisher, J. C. (2002). A nationwide study of the influence of faculty development programs on colleague relationships. *Academic Medicine* 77(5): 402–406. doi: 10.1097/00001888-200205000-00010.

Nelson, D. J., and Rogers, D. C. (2003). A national analysis of diversity in science and engineering faculties at research universities. Washington, DC: National Organization for Women.

Odom, K. L., Roberts, L. M., Johnson, R. L., and Cooper, L. A. (2007). Exploring obstacles to and opportunities for professional success among ethnic minority medical students. *Academic Medicine* 82(2): 146–153. doi: 10.1097/acm.0b013e31802d8f2c.

Pfeffer, J., Fong, C. T., Cialdini, R. B., and Portnoy, R. R. (2006). Overcoming the self-promotion dilemma: Interpersonal attraction and extra help as a consequence of who sings one's praises. *Personality and Social Psychology Bulletin* 32(10): 1362–1374. doi: 10.1177/0146167206290337.

Ross-Smith, A., and Chesterman, C. (2009). "Girl disease": Women managers' reticence and ambivalence toward organizational advancement. *Journal of Management & Organization* 15(5): 582–595. doi: 10.5172/jmo.15.5.582.

Rudman, L. A. (1998). Self-promotion as a risk factor for women: The costs and benefits of counterstereotypical impression management. *Journal of Personality and Social Psychology* 74(3): 629–645. doi: 10.1037//0022-3514.74.3.629.

Scopelliti, I., Loewenstein, G., and Vosgerau, J. (2015). You call it "self-exuberance," I call it bragging: Miscalibrated predictions of emotional responses to self-promotion. *Psychological Science* 26(6): 903–214. doi: 10.1177/0956797615573516.

Sloma-Williams, L., McDade, S. A., Richman, R. C., Morahan, P. S., Dean, D., Bracken, S., et al. (2009). The role of self-efficacy in developing women leaders. In *Women in Academic Leadership: Professional Strategies, Personal Choices* (pp. 50–73). Sterling, VA: Stylus.

Sue, D. W., Capodilupo, C. M., Torino, G. C., Bucceri, J. M., Holder, A. M., Nadal, K. L., and Esquilin, M. (2007). Racial microaggressions in everyday life: Implications for clinical practice. *American Psychologist*, 62(4): 271–286. doi: 10.1037/0003-066x.62.4.271.

White, F. S., McDade, S., Yamagata, H., and Morahan, P. S. (2012). Gender-related differences in the pathway to and characteristics of U.S. medical school deanships. *Academic Medicine* 87(8): 1015–1023. doi: 10.1097/acm.0b013e31825d3495.

Wright, A. L., Schwindt, L. A., Bassford, T. L., Reyna, V. F., Shisslak, C. M., Germain, P. A., and Reed, K. L. (2003). Gender differences in academic advancement. *Academic Medicine* 78(5): 500–508. doi: 10.1097/00001888-200305000-00015.

Zea, M. C., Jarama, S. L., and Bianchi, F. T. (1995). Social support and psychosocial competence: Explaining the adaptation to college of ethnically diverse students. *American Journal of Community Psychology* 23(4): 509–531. doi: 10.1007/bf02506966.

SECTION II

Professionalism Issues

6

Teaching Women and Minorities

The Challenges of Microaggressions in Medical Education

DIANNE GOEDE, DANIELLE PANNA,
ZAREEN ZAIDI, AND MONICA VELA[1]

Aequitas enim lucet ipsa per se—Equity shines by her own light.

Cicero

In this chapter we define the term "microaggressions" and provide a literature review on the impact of microaggressions on female and minority learners and faculty. We provide strategies on an individual and institutional level to deal with microaggressions.

Objectives

Define the term "microaggressions."
Identify microaggressions in medical education.
Analyze the psychological toll of microaggressions on female and minority learners and faculty.
Identify strategies to deal with microaggressions.

"Wait, who are you?" The male veteran asked the female resident standing before him. She was dressed professionally, in dress pants, a blouse and white coat with her ID badge visibly displayed with the title "Doctor" in bold print under her photo. The resident had just finished introducing herself to the patient who was in the emergency room waiting for admission.

---

1   Dianne Goede, M.D., University of Florida College of Medicine, Gainesville, FL.
Danielle Panna, M.D., University of Florida College of Medicine, Gainesville, FL.
Zareen Zaidi, M.D., Ph.D., University of Florida College of Medicine, Gainesville, FL.
Monica Vela, M.D., Pritzker School of Medicine, Chicago, IL.

She again stated her title and the patient responded, "No, I just spoke with my doctor, he came in before you." She clarified to the patient that the man who just exited the room was a new nurse just coming on shift and she was indeed his doctor. The patient flushed and said, "OK, well I don't understand why I need to keep repeating myself." The resident nodded and proceeded to perform the history and physical examination.

"I am not going to take that medicine, it makes me sick and I will not take it. How do I know that I can even trust him anyway?" The medicine ward team listened as their 50-year-old male Caucasian Iraq war veteran patient pointed to an American-born male intern of Asian ethnicity to express skepticism over the medical treatment provided. It was halfway through the internship year and the intern was working tirelessly on the Internal Medicine in-patient service.

Despite making some strides in enrollment to medical schools in recent years, women and minorities continue to be poorly represented in leadership or senior positions (Bickel et al. 2002; Morahan et al. 2011; Orom et al. 2013). According to the Association of American Medical Colleges (AAMC): women comprise 47 percent of matriculants to medical school, but make up only 21 percent of full professors and 16 percent of deans as of 2013–2014 (AAMC 2008; Lautenberger et al. 2014). The number of minorities who have successfully traversed the pipeline into the academic medical profession is also low. An analysis of medical school faculty confirms that minorities comprise only 4 percent of faculty positions nationally (Betancourt 2006). Senior leadership positions such as dean or chair also lack diversity: 4 percent African Americans, 5 percent Asian Americans, and 5 percent Hispanic (Mader et al. 2016). A recent survey studied the sex of grand round speakers in nine specialties and found that the representation of women falls below the percentage of women medical students (47 percent) and is lower than women faculty (36 percent) (Boiko et al. 2017). Research has shown that minorities and women have made progress in academic medicine from 1997 to 2008, but at such a slow pace that "at current rate, it would take nearly 1,000 years for the proportion of African American physicians to catch up to the percentage of African Americans in the general population" (Yu et al. 2013, p. 212).

In the United States, underrepresented minorities make up 15 percent of total medical school enrollment (Castillo-Page 2015). This enrollment level is in sharp contrast to the 31 percent of the current U.S. population identified as racial or cultural minorities (U.S. Census Bureau 2016). Boatright et al. (2017) explored the influence of race on Alpha Omega Alpha election among applicants to Yale residency programs and found that Alpha Omega Alpha membership for white students was nearly six times greater than that for African American students and nearly two times greater than Asian students. Studies have cited negative experiences and lack of role models as reasons for the "leakiness of the pipeline"—that is, departure of students from the path to a medical or dental profession (Freeman et al. 2016. Dark-skinned women often claim that they are discounted on the basis of their skin color, sex, or both (Cooke 2017). The landscape of medical professionals is discordant with the general population of the United States. According to the U.S. Census Bureau, nonwhites will make up 56 percent of the population in 2060: Hispanics/Latinos, 28 percent; African Americans, 14 percent; Asians Americans, 9 percent; American Indian and Alaska Native, 1.3 percent; and mixed races, 6 percent (Colby and Ortman 2015; U.S. Census Bureau 2016).

Sexual and gender minorities are also poorly represented. A recent survey sent out across the United States and Canada (M.D. and D.O. schools) reported a total of 912 sexual minority students and 35 gender minority individuals enrolled from 2009 to 2010 (Mansh et al. 2015). Many participants in the survey concealed their identities, citing a fear of discrimination (42 percent) and lack of support. This in turn has significant negative effects on physical and mental well-being. First-year sexual minority medical students experience significantly greater risk of anxiety and depression secondary to harassment and isolation (Przedworski et al. 2015). A survey of heterosexual medical students found that nearly half (48 percent) reported explicit bias, and 81 percent of students demonstrated implicit bias toward gay men and lesbian women (Nadal et al. 2016). To provide effective health care to this rapidly changing population, it is imperative that we train future doctors to be sensitive to this increasingly culturally diverse population (Hamilton 2009).

Diversity in medical education is critical if we are to address the health and health care disparities so prevalent among minority populations. Studies have shown that diversity in the medical profession benefits patients by providing more choices, better access to health care for minority patients, and higher patient satisfaction, while also providing an improved educational experience for health professions students (Perez et al. 2007). In addition, learners who are taught diversity through exposure in medi-

cal school report improved preparedness to take care of diverse populations (Boutin-Foster et al. 2008; Lopez et al. 2008). Medical schools have
increased their effort to recruit faculty members of underrepresented
minorities, but need to ensure that those minorities have positive experiences in school in order to maintain the pipeline of minority students,
faculty, and leaders in academic medicine (Bickel et al. 2002).

Given the importance of diversity in medical education, we require
an analysis of the reasons behind the discordance of the demographics
in academic medicine. Frequently identified barriers for the advancement of women in academic medicine and a lack of retention of women
in academic medicine (the "leaky pipeline") include a disproportionate
burden of family responsibilities, lack of gender equality in compensation, and lack of parity in pay and leadership by gender (Carr et al. 2015).
Reports describe up to 70 percent of female faculty reporting gender-
based discrimination, with 48 percent of female physicians reporting
sexist comments and 30 percent reporting severe harassment (compared
to 3 percent of male colleagues) (Carr et al. 2003; Carr et al. 2015). Carr
et al. (2015) found that women physicians who experienced gender discrimination reported lower self-confidence and self-esteem and tended
to become isolated in academic institutions. Studies have documented
that even though men and women residents may receive similar evaluations at the beginning of residency, a gender gap in evaluations continues
until graduation (Dayal et al. 2017). Other challenges faced by minorities
include racism—per one report, 20 percent of medical students and 23
percent of residents in the United States have experiences racism and discrimination (Beagan 2003). Minority medical students who experience
discrimination and stereotype threats during their education and training
often feel significant pressure to dispel negative stereotypes and represent
their entire race or culture (Chandauka et al. 2015; Dickins et al. 2013;
Odom et al. 2007). They may feel that their race has an adverse effect on
their ability to seek academic and social support in medical school (Sánchez et al. 2013). Financial barriers, lack of social support, challenges with
standardized tests, and experiences with racial stereotyping are just some
of the barriers identified (Odom et al. 2007; Orom et al. 2013). Because a
negative climate leads women and minorities to underperform—which
may result in discouragement, dropping out, and a loss in the workforce—
it is imperative that institutions and educators work to enhance the cli-

mate for diversity, improve cultural awareness, and employ strategies to reduce biases among all stakeholders (Steele 2011). The chapter on Graceful Self-Promotion in this book provides further insights into individual and institutional measures that can prevent attrition of women and minorities in the workforce.

Conceptual Framework

The conceptual framework of this chapter is based on Sue's (2010) work on microaggressions. Below is a definition of the term followed by detailed examples:

> The term "microaggression" refers to "everyday subtle put downs directed towards a marginalized group which may be verbal or nonverbal and are typically automatic." Microaggressions send disparaging messages to individuals because of their group of membership. Often the perpetrators of microaggressions are not aware of their actions. (Sue 2010, p. 5)

Microaggressions are a less visible modern form of racism. In contrast to the overt "old-fashioned" racism, microaggression is an "ambiguous and nebulous form that is more difficult to identify" (Sue 2010, p. 23). It is a mechanism by which gender and racial bias persists. Microaggressions can be carried out through subtle exchanges, looks, or gestures in a pattern that devalues race or gender, often without any actual intention by the perpetrator (Sue et al. 2007). While the examples we provide in this chapter focus on women and racial minorities, it is important to note that other ethnic minorities, sexual and gender minorities, and people with disabilities also encounter microaggressions.

In the health care profession, women and minority physicians often need to clarify their titles as they are mistaken for nurses or other service providers. The underlying message conveyed is that you must not be a doctor because you are a woman or minority. Such messages take a mental tax on the victims over time, which is addressed ahead.

Sue et al. identify three categories of microaggressions: microinsults, microassaults, and microinvalidations (2007). Whereas microassaults, such as outright racist statements or acts, are typically consciously committed by a perpetrator, microinsults and microinvalidations are usually

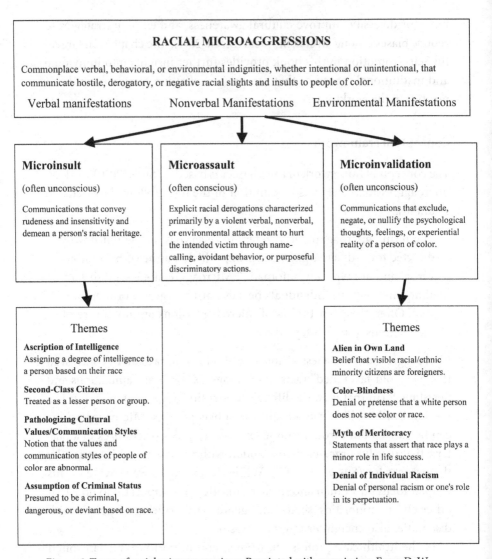

Figure 6. Types of racial microaggressions. Reprinted with permission. From D. W. Sue, *Microaggressions in everyday life: Race, gender, and sexual orientation* (Hoboken, NJ: Wiley, 2010). Copyright © 2010 by John Wiley & Sons, Inc. All rights reserved.

unconscious. Given that overt microassaults are unacceptable in society, medical students, residents, medical faculty, and other allied health professionals who are members of a marginalized group are more likely to experience microinvalidations and microinsults. Figure 6 provides a summary of the three forms of microaggressions.

Microinsults

An African American pulmonary critical care fellow in her last year of fellowship described an encounter with a white patient she was admitting to the hospital. Prior to entering the room, a male medical student and male resident (both white) had examined the patient. She entered the room to supervise the encounter, confirm physical exam findings, and discuss the plan of care with the patient. She wore medical scrubs and a white coat. Before she introduced herself, the patient held up his hand and said, "Oh, no, they have already come in to take my lunch order, thank you." The doctor was stunned. She corrected the patient and told him she was his doctor and supervised the two men who had just left the room. The patient was flustered and embarrassed. He apologized for his statement. The doctor completed her exam, and left the room to rejoin the group.

Microinsults are most often conveyed as subtle cut-downs hidden in interpersonal communication or in the environment that convey stereotypes and demean a person's racial, gender, or sexual orientation or heritage (Sue 2010). Comments that are unconsciously disguised as a compliment or a positive statement may in fact be a "put-down" comment. Forms of microinsults include:

Ascription of intelligence: Assigning intelligence to a person on the basis of race—for example, telling African Americans that they are a credit to their race, or assuming that all Asians are intelligent or good at math.

Second-class citizen: Treating a person as a lesser person—for example, mistaking a person of color for a service person, ignoring a person of color in a white crowd, or mistaking a woman health care professional for a nurse.

Pathologizing cultural communication: The notion that the communication style of a person of color is abnormal—for example, telling African Americans that they are loud or Asians that they too quiet. This also sends a message that minorities should assimilate to the dominant culture.

Assumption of criminal status: Presuming that a person of color, specifically an African American, is a criminal—for example, a store owner following a person of color around a store, or casting suspicious glances at a person of color in a public area (Sue et al. 2007).

Microassaults

A third-year woman medical student rotating on a colorectal surgery service presented a patient outside the patient's room to the other members of the team, who were men. The patient was an elderly female presenting with rectal prolapse. As a part of the history, the medical student mentioned that the patient also had uterine prolapse and used a pessary device, which remained in place at the time of examination. The fellow asked the surgical intern what a pessary device was. The intern did not know the answer. The female medical student stated, "A pessary is a plastic device placed in the vagina to help treat the symptoms of uterine prolapse." The male fellow turned to the student and said, "Oh? How would you know? Do you use one?" The male surgical resident and intern laughed. The medical student quipped, "Yes, daily." The team went in to see the patient.

A microassault is a deliberate, conscious attack directed at a marginalized group that may be subtle or explicit. They are racial-, gender-, or sexual-orientation–biased attitudes, behaviors, or beliefs that are communicated through environmental cues, verbalizations, or behaviors (Sue 2010). In contrast to microinsults and microinvalidations, perpetrators committing microassaults harbor a conscious bias expressed as racist statements/behavior, sexist comments, or heterosexism.

The above example is a microassault on the medical student's gender. Prior to that moment, she had felt like a member of the team. However, by making these comments, the men on the team had alienated the student. During the third year of medical school, medical students begin to select their specialty interests as they are exposed to different fields in clerkships. In a longitudinal study of female medical students, negative gendered experiences encountered during third-year clerkships impacted students' choice of subspecialty (Babaria and Nunez-Smith 2009). The student described coped with the situation by minimalizing it and replying with a joke. Unfortunately, incidents like these impact self-esteem and often career choices.

Microinvalidations

A faculty member walks into her patient's room in the clinic. The patient asks the doctor, "Where are you from?" The doctor politely answers that she was born in Iran. The patient then looks incredulously at her dress and asks, "Do they let you dress like that there?" The faculty member attempts to steer the discussion back toward the patient and the patient's chief complaint. Nonetheless, the doctor is left uncomfortable.

Microinvalidations represent the most damaging of the three types of microaggressions. They deny the racial, gender, or sexual orientation reality of the marginalized groups they are directed toward and shift their experiential reality. The metacommunication or hidden messages during such encounters leave minorities feeling as if they were not from the country they were living in and serving and that they were foreign, and therefore unwelcome. Unfortunately, microinvalidations permeate medical training landscapes. Forms of microinvalidation include:

Alien in One's Own Land: The assumption that Asian Americans, Latinos, or other racial minorities are foreign-born. Repeated comments like "Where are you from?" or "You speak English well" are examples.

Color blindness: The unwillingness to admit to seeing race or a person's color. Comments like "I don't see color when I look at people" or "The most qualified person should get the job, regardless of color or background" are typical examples and exhibit a denial of the role of power and privilege.

Myth of meritocracy: Implying that people of color are benefiting from their race.

Denial of individual racism: Statements made by whites such as "I have several black friends" or "I am a woman, so I understand your race issues" are attempts to deny racial bias (Sue 2010).

A female medical student rose to the podium at an internal medicine conference to give an oral case presentation. Rather than a "traditional" oral presentation, she presented her case as a sonnet. It had all the required elements of an oral presentation, and it flowed well. The audience perked up and leaned in to listen. The presenter gained confidence as she progressed through her presentation and once she finished, she smiled. She took a seat to answer questions from the judges. One judge prefaced his question with a comment, "your presentation was cute, by the way."

In this example, the student's unique and thoughtful presentation of an interesting medical case was cut down to something that was "cute." She had gained confidence from her presentation, and began to feel a part of the established group of physicians surrounding her. Although the judge never intended to cause harm, his comment that her presentation was "cute" was derogatory and nullified her accomplishments as a professional.

The Psychological Toll of Microaggressions

A woman resident interested in a career in critical care is excited for her first ICU rotation. She is eager to shine and make a positive impression. She is well prepared for daily rounds. When the team arrives at the bedside of her patients, she begins her presentation. To her surprise, the male fellow interrupts her presentation and won't allow her to present her assessment and plan. She is embarrassed and assumes she is doing a poor job, so she alters her presentation style. She asks the attending physician and fellow for feedback on her performance and they tell her she is doing a good job and to keep up the good work. After a week, she notices the fellow does not interrupt her male resident counterpart during his presentations. Daily on rounds, she is distracted by the different treatment that is shown to her male counterpart and slowly she grows frustrated. By the end of the rotation, she is exhausted from trying to attain equal treatment and respect on the team and finds herself questioning her desire to seek a critical care fellowship.

During a typical four-year medical school curriculum, the first two years include early-clinical exposure to patients, but it is the third year when medical students are deployed to the hospital wards, where they immerse themselves in clinical medicine and patient care. Paralleling this clinical experience, they also experience the hidden curriculum of medical education. This hidden curriculum teaches them how to model the behaviors expected of a doctor. They learn through observing their attending physicians and residents in the clinical environment. The medical student has both direct encounters with these mentors and indirect encounters, where they observe behaviors and slowly adapt to function in the clinical environment. It is often as part of the hidden curriculum that students, especially those who have been historically underrepresented in medicine such as minorities and woman, begin experiencing microaggressions that will shape their careers. An institution's hidden curriculum impacts not just students but trainees and faculty. Therefore, paying attention to the hidden institutional culture can impact perceptions of individuals from different social groups. Increased interracial contact and curricula focusing on cultural awareness can also impact attitudes (Saha et al. 2008; Taylor and Rust 1999; van Ryn et al. 2015).

Microaggressions demonstrating gender discrimination take a heavy toll on female physicians. Female physician faculty members who experienced gender discrimination feel a loss of professional self-confidence and develop cynicism toward their profession. The loss of self-confidence leads to decreased interest in undergoing the scrutiny of the academic promotion process (Carr et al. 2003). In academic medicine, the targets for promotion are elusive and constantly redefined by those in leadership. Most of those in leadership are male, and thus woman perceive there is a lack of support for their advancement. This perception dampens motivational drive for advancement, since many women learn to view it as an uphill and exhausting battle. The phrase "death by a thousand cuts" or "a ton of feathers" best describes how the cumulative toll of microaggressions experienced daily by female and minority physicians slowly erodes their ambitions and goals (Carr et al. 2003).

When taken as isolated events, one might dismiss microaggressions as unfortunate events unlikely to cause detriment to the victim. However, these common daily experiences of aggression may have a more significant influence on anger, frustration, and self-esteem than traditional overt forms of racism, sexism, and heterosexism (Sue 2010). It is the cumulative effects of microaggressions on self-esteem and frustration levels that lead to the well-documented "leaky pipeline" for women and minorities, particularly in academic medicine (Ash et al. 2004).

Given that microaggressions signify a hostile environment, it is understandable that the victims develop maladaptive behaviors. Depression, hypervigilance, skepticism, rage, anger, fatigue, and hopelessness all may be experienced by the victims of microaggressions (Sue 2010). In a longitudinal study of medical students spanning the third-year medical curriculum, female medical students became desensitized to inappropriate behaviors and noted that they were "just too tired to care" (Babaria et al. 2012, p. 1018). Decreased self-confidence, cynicism, and anger are other signs of the cumulative effects of microaggressions.

When female and minority medical students experience microaggressions, their cognitive skills suffer. A study documented the cognitive functions of minority and white persons before and after exposing them to both subtle and overt examples of racial bias. Minorities showed a decline in cognitive functioning after examples of subtle bias, whereas white persons showed a decline in cognitive functioning after they were shown overt examples of racial bias (Salvatore and Shelton 2007). Subtle bias is often difficult to discern, and may distract the mental faculties of the victim. In an academic setting, students' attention is diverted from their studies while they attempt to discern if a microaggression truly occurred or if they are being overly sensitive. When studied, minority medical students experienced race-related discrimination and other race-related experiences at a much high frequency than their nonminority colleagues. Minority medical students are more likely to express a lower satisfaction with their learning environment compared with white students. Minority students have lower USMLE scores and GPAs than their white colleagues and are more likely to experience graduation delays and failure in medical school (Orom et al. 2013). Minorities also tend to have a lower sense of personal accomplishment and lower scores on quality-of-life surveys (Dyrbye et al. 2006a): with women medical students experiencing more psychological distress (Blanch et al. 2008; Dyrbye 2006b).

Strategies to Move Forward

Individual

We ask our readers to pause for a moment before reading on and think about how they would respond in the following situations (keeping in mind the earlier scenarios):

Should the woman medical student respond to the insinuation about her using pessaries?

What should the African American critical care fellow do after her interaction with the patient who thought she was a food service worker?

How should the woman medical student respond to the judge's comment that her presentation was "cute"?

The decision to react or not is an important decision, described as a "Catch-22" dilemma or "damned if you do and damned if you don't" situation by Sue et al. (2007). Very often in the spur of the moment, recipients may not be able to determine if the incident is a microaggression. Even if they correctly identify a microaggression, they may adopt a form of denial or simply not know how to respond. Additionally, a fear of repercussion may prevent them from speaking up (Sue et al. 2007). Most institutions have a mechanism for reporting microassaults, as these usually are blatant racist statements or actions. Although little research evidence exists regarding coping strategies to deal with microinvalidations and microinsults specifically in health professions education, a summary of some strategies described in the literature are provided below:

> *Providing "counterspaces"* is essential for the academic success of minority students, according to studies (Grier-Reed 2010; Solorzano et al. 2000). Counterspaces are intentionally created networks, safe spaces, or sanctuaries where participants can develop relationships and support for coping with microaggressions. Researchers define them as "sites where deficit notions of people of color can be challenged and where a positive collegiate racial climate can be established and maintained" (Solorzano et al. 2000, p. 70), spaces that help participants develop a positive cultural identity (Brondolo et al. 2009). African American, Latino, Asian American, or LGBT groups are all examples of counterspaces. In these groups, participants can express themselves in a nonjudgmental environment. They can also draw on the collective wisdom of the crowd in deciding how to respond to microaggressions. Studies have found that social support is an important factor in determining academic success with research at the collegiate level: students who talked to others about their perceptions of being treated unfairly had a higher grade point average then those who did not talk to others (Zea et al. 1995). Social networks have also been noted to have a positive impact on building resilience (Burdick 2014).
>
> *Verbalizing the issue*, confronting, or educating others are strategies that minorities can use if appropriate (Hernández et al. 2010). Krieger and Sidney (1996) found that these strategies decrease blood pressure in students exposed to microaggressions, whereas an "avoidant coping mechanism" may exacerbate stress (West et

al. 2009). Greene and Blitz (2011) examined conveying a message using humor, a strategy that may be particularly useful with interracial dialogue training.

Seeking out mentors for advice in such situations is imperative (Dobkin and Hutchinson 2013; Hernández et al. 2010). Formal mentoring programs have been shown to increase group cohesion, and result in both greater progress of the mentees and an increase in the number of ethnic minority staff (Buddeberg-Fischer and Herta 2006). Mentors can help strategize how to respond to microaggressions and may have a role in decision-making processes, therefore championing policy changes on the behalf of the mentee. It is of note that the ability of male faculty to effectively mentor women depends on their understanding of the challenges faced by women. Skilled mentors can achieve a greater impact in a limited time period (Bickel 2014).

Becoming involved in social action—for example, joining or starting a group; writing or researching to create awareness; petitioning leadership to improve institutional climate—is a positive coping strategy (Laird et al. 2005).

Practicing mindfulness reduces stress and anxiety in medical students (Hassed et al. 2009; Rosenzweig et al. 2003; Warnecke et al. 2011) as well as health care professionals (Epstein and Krasner 2013; Irving et al. 2009). Epstein (1999) describes mindful medical practice as an extension of reflective practice, helping the practitioner to become "more aware of one's own mental processes, listen more attentively, become flexible, and recognize bias and judgment, and thereby act with principles and compassion" (p. 835). Breathing exercises, yoga, meditation, guided imagery, art, and narrative medicine are some useful techniques (Dobkin and Hutchinson 2013).

Tapping spirituality and using prayer and rituals can also help minorities cope with frustrations brought up by microaggressions (Koenig et al. 2010; Rosenzweig et al. 2003).

Institutional

It is important that institutions own their role in creating systems that support continued systemic racism, discrimination, unconscious bias, and microaggressions. While the recommendations made above address the importance of caring for those exposed to these detrimental mechanisms, institutions also need to build mechanisms that encourage a positive diverse climate, and that allow for cultural humility and harmony among all students, staff, and faculty. Studies have repeatedly challenged the institutional "color-blind" and often passive approach to promoting diversity (Sue et al. 2007). Ignoring racial and gender identities places minority groups at a disadvantage in recruitment, retention, and promotion (Bickel et al. 2002; Sue 2010). Below is a summary of the recommendation by Sue (2010) for institutions to overcome systematic bias:

Creating forums or hosting focus groups to hear the voices of individuals of color, women, and LGBT prevents them from feeling isolated and devalued. Supporting and nourishing minority meetings and groups on campus or at an institution increases multicultural interaction, provides a support system, and sends a strong message about the organizational climate.

Positive role modeling by leadership promotes a bias-free work environment, with the understanding that we all have inherent biases and need training to gain insights into our own biases.

Meaningful vision statements with objective action plans addressing disparities can create a welcoming environment.

An oversight team/group empowered to assess, develop, and monitor the organization's multicultural initiatives is essential.

The leadership at all levels (dean to division heads) must be held accountable for recruiting, retaining, and promoting minorities.

Additional recommendations include:

The institution must make a long-term commitment to educate and train students, staff, and faculty on implicit bias at all levels and on an ongoing basis. One tool that can be used to create awareness of biases is the "Implicit Association Test" (IAT, available free online), which measures attitudes and beliefs that people may be unwilling or unable to report (Green et al. 2007). Such exercises should be followed by debriefing meetings and advanced training opportunities.

Institutions should develop longitudinal curricula that focus on diversity training, utilizing multiple teaching formats including:

lectures, seminars, and workshops; communication skills training; community-based learning involving field work; and e-learning using blogs, online lectures, webinars, and videos. In planning these curricula, institutions must pay special attention to the following areas to illustrate diversity issues: groups with disabilities; social deprivation; gender; sexuality; ethnicity; age; marginalized groups, for example, the homeless or refugees (Dogra et al. 2016).

Returning to the Scenarios

Should the woman medical student respond to the insinuation about her using pessaries? Empowering women to speak up is important. However, she should first assess the power dynamic, the potential for retaliation, and the potential for a positive outcome. Often, students will need to reach out to diversity officers or deans for advice. Students may need to wait for evaluations to be submitted before asking for a word in private with the senior resident to verbalize their concerns.

What should the African American critical care fellow do after her interaction with the patient who thought she was the nurse? Here, the fellow already explained that she was a doctor to the patient, so engaging further in a conversation with the patient would not be helpful. Again, assessing the potential for change and the impact on ongoing relationships is important. As situations like these lead to rumination and later anxiety and depression, a support group is helpful. If she is involved with an African American support group or has a faculty mentor, she should discuss the situation.

How should the woman medical student respond to the judge's comment that her presentation was "cute"? Here again the student could confront the judge about his use of the word "cute" to describe her work. An even better outcome would result if another judge, male or female, were to step in to provide a constructive assessment of her performance, thereby both providing role modeling to the first judge, and remedying some of the impact of the microaggression.

Final Thoughts

Educators must remain vigilant of the multifaceted challenges learners face during their medical education. Women and minority medical students face a very convoluted set of challenges as they navigate the choppy waters of medical training. As described above, the automatic everyday put-downs they experience, either in verbal or nonverbal, forms have cumulative psychological effects. In addition to anxiety and depression, microaggressions lead to poor performance secondary to lack of confidence, a feeling of worthlessness, loss of drive, and paranoia (D'Andrea and Daniels 2007). Unfortunately, a vast body of literature demonstrates the association between racial discrimination and poor health outcomes (Wong et al. 2014). Depression, anxiety, hypertension, cardiovascular, pulmonary, and pain conditions are reported more commonly in minorities (Gee et al. 2007a; Gee et al. 2007b; Harrell et al. 2003; Herek 2009; Mays et al. 2007). The emotional dysregulation created by stress can result in increased rumination, impulsive behavior, and even substance abuse problems (Blume et al. 2012; Hatzenbuehler et al. 2009).

Learners often choose to ignore microaggressions and assume they will eventually cease. While avoidance is a coping strategy, there are many other strategies that we must teach women and minority learners. Additionally, institutions must put in place mechanisms to improve the environment for these learners. These institutional mechanisms are not only important to advocate for improving the resilience of women and minorities, but to remove harmful practices at institutional levels.

Questions for Future Research

In this era of global turmoil, immigration issues, and terrorism, it is particularly important that we develop institutional policies and programs to support diversity and create cultural awareness. The National Science Foundation's ADVANCE awards (advancement of women in academic science and engineering careers) are one model. The program for transformational culture change in academic institutions regarding advancement of women in science, technology, engineering, and mathematics (STEM) fields is an example of a longitudinal program that addresses individual, institutional, and national needs (Laursen et al. 2015). Further research is suggested:

As institutions develop longitudinal programs to support culture change and diversity, they need research data to provide "how to" guidelines for developing such initiatives.

As programs evolve, researchers must focus on developing evaluations to document the impact of such programs.

References

Ash, A. S., Carr, P. L., Goldstein, R., and Friedman, R. H. (2004). Compensation and advancement of women in academic medicine: Is there equity? *Annals of Internal Medicine* 141(3): 205. doi: 10.7326/0003-4819-141-3-200408030-00009.

Association of American Medical Colleges (AAMC). (2008). *U.S. medical school applicants and students, 1982–1983 to 2007–2008*. Retrieved April 6, 2017, from https://www.aamc.org/data/facts/enrollmentgraduate/158808/total-enrollment-by-medical-school-by-sex.html.

Babaria, P., Abedin, S., Berg, D., and Nunez-Smith, M. (2012). "I'm too used to it": A longitudinal qualitative study of third year female medical students' experiences of gendered encounters in medical education. *Social Science & Medicine* 74(7): 1013–1020. doi: 10.1016/j.socscimed.2011.11.043.

Babaria, P., Abedin, S., and Nunez-Smith, M. (2009). The effect of gender on the clinical clerkship experiences of female medical students: Results from a qualitative study. *Academic Medicine* 84(7): 859–866. doi: 10.1097/acm.0b013e3181a8130c.

Beagan, B. L. (2003). "Is this worth getting into a big fuss over?" Everyday racism in medical school. *Medical Education* 37(10): 852–860. doi: 10.1046/j.1365-2923.2003.01622.x.

Betancourt, J. R. (2006). Eliminating racial and ethnic disparities in health care: What is the role of academic medicine? *Academic Medicine* 81(9): 788–792. doi: 10.1097/00001888-200609000-00004.

Bickel, J. (2014). How men can excel as mentors of women. *Academic Medicine* 89(8): 1100–1102. doi: 10.1097/acm.0000000000000313.

Bickel, J., Wara, D., Atkinson, B. F., Cohen, L. S., Dunn, M., Hostler, S., et al. (2002). Increasing women's leadership in academic medicine: Report of the AAMC project implementation committee. *Academic Medicine* 77(10): 1043–1061. doi: 10.1097/00001888-200210000-00023.

Blanch, D. C., Hall, J. A., Roter, D. L., and Frankel, R. M. (2008). Medical student gender and issues of confidence. *Patient Education and Counseling* 72(3): 374–381. doi: 10.1016/j.pec.2008.05.021.

Blume, A. W., Lovato, L. V., Thyken, B. N., and Denny, N. (2012). The relationship of microaggressions with alcohol use and anxiety among ethnic minority college students in a historically White institution. *Cultural Diversity and Ethnic Minority Psychology* 18(1): 45–54. doi: 10.1037/a0025457.

Boatright, D., Ross, D., O'Connor, P., Moore, E., and Nunez-Smith, M. (2017, May). Racial disparities in medical student membership in the Alpha Omega Alpha Honor Society. *JAMA Internal Medicine* 177(5):659–665. doi: 10.1001/jamainternmed.2016.9623.

Boiko, J. R., Anderson, A. J., and Gordon, R. A. (2017, May). Representation of women among academic grand rounds speakers. *JAMA Internal Medicine* 177(5): 722–724. doi: 10.1001/jamainternmed.2016.9646.

Boutin-Foster, C., Foster, J. C., and Konopasek, L. (2008). Viewpoint: Physician, know thyself: The professional culture of medicine as a framework for teaching cultural competence. *Academic Medicine* 83(1): 106–111. doi: 10.1097/acm.0b013e31815c6753.

Brondolo, E., Halen, N. B., Pencille, M., Beatty, D., and Contrada, R. J. (2009). Coping with racism: A selective review of the literature and a theoretical and methodological critique. *Journal of Behavioral Medicine* 32(1): 64–88. doi: 10.1007/s10865-008-9193-0.

Buddeberg-Fischer, B., and Herta, K. (2006). Formal mentoring programmes for medical students and doctors—a review of the Medline literature. *Medical Teacher* 28(3): 248–257. doi: 10.1080/01421590500313043.

Burdick, W. P. (2014). Social networks (and more) are necessary for student and faculty resilience. *Medical Education* 49(1): 17–19. doi: 10.1111/medu.12607.

Carr, P. L., Gunn, C. M., Kaplan, S. A., Raj, A., and Freund, K. M. (2015). Inadequate progress for women in academic medicine: Findings from the National Faculty Study. *Journal of Women's Health* 24(3): 190–199. doi: 10.1089/jwh.2014.4848.

Carr, P. L., Szalacha, L., Barnett, R., Caswell, C., and Inui, T. (2003). A "ton of feathers": Gender discrimination in academic medical careers and how to manage it. *Journal of Women's Health* 12(10): 1009–1018. doi: 10.1089/154099903322643938.

Castillo-Page, L. (2015). *Diversity in medical education: Facts & figures 2012.* Retrieved April 3, 2017, from https://members.aamc.org/eweb/upload/Diversity%20in%20Medical%20Education_Facts%20and%20Figures%202012.pdf.

Chandauka, R. E., Russell, J. M., Sandars, J., and Vivekananda-Schmidt, P. (2015). Differing perceptions among ethnic minority and Caucasian medical students which may affect their relative academic performance. *Education for Primary Care* 26(1): 11–15. doi: 10.1080/14739879.2015.11494301.

Colby, S. L., and Ortman, J. M. (2015). *Projections of the size and composition of the U.S. population: 2014 to 2060.* Washington, DC: U.S. Census Bureau.

Cooke, M. (2017, May). Implicit bias in academic medicine. *JAMA Internal Medicine.* 177(5):657–658. doi: 10.1001/jamainternmed.2016.9643.

D'Andrea, M., and Daniels, J. (2007). Dealing with institutional racism on campus: Initiating difficult dialogues and social justice advocacy interventions. *College Student Affairs Journal* 26(2): 169–176.

Dayal, A., O'Connor, D. M., Qadri, U., and Arora, V. M. (2017, May). Comparison of male vs female resident milestone evaluations by faculty during emergency medicine residency training. *JAMA Internal Medicine* 177(5): 651–657. doi: 10.1001/jamainternmed.2016.9616.

Dickins, K., Levinson, D., Smith, S. G., and Humphrey, H. J. (2013). The minority student voice at one medical school. *Academic Medicine* 88(1): 73–79. doi: 10.1097/acm.0b013e3182769513.

Dobkin, P. L., and Hutchinson, T. A. (2013). Teaching mindfulness in medical school: Where are we now and where are we going? *Medical Education* 47(8): 768–779. doi: 10.1111/medu.12200.

Dogra, N., Bhatti, F., Ertubey, C., Kelly, M., Rowlands, A., Singh, D., et al. (2016). Teaching diversity to medical undergraduates: Curriculum development, delivery and assessment. AMEE GUIDE no. 103. *Medical Teacher* 38(4): 323–337. doi: 10.3109/0142159X.2015.1105944.

Dyrbye, L. N., Thomas, M. R., Huschka, M. M., Lawson, K. L., Novotny, P. J., Sloan, J. A., and Shanafelt, T. D. (2006a). A multicenter study of burnout, depression, and quality of life in minority and nonminority U.S. medical students. *Mayo Clinic Proceedings* 81(11): 1435–1442. doi: 10.4065/81.11.1435.

Dyrbye, L. N., Thomas, M. R., and Shanafelt, T. D. (2006b). Systematic review of depression, anxiety, and other indicators of psychological distress among U.S. and Canadian medical students. *Academic Medicine* 81(4): 354–373. doi: 10.1097/00001888-200604000-00009.

Epstein, R. M. (1999). Mindful practice. *JAMA* 282(9): 833–839. doi: 10.1001/jama .282.9.833.

Epstein, R. M., and Krasner, M. S. (2013). Physician resilience: What it means, why it matters, and how to promote it. *Academic Medicine* 88(3): 301–303. doi: 10.1097/ acm.0b013e318280cff0.

Freeman, B. K., Landry, A., Trevino, R., Grande, D., and Shea, J. A. (2016). Understanding the leaky pipeline. *Academic Medicine* 91(7): 987–993. doi: 10.1097/acm .0000000000001020.

Gee, G. C., Spencer, M. S., Chen, J., and Takeuchi, D. (2007a). A nationwide study of discrimination and chronic health conditions among Asian Americans. *American Journal of Public Health* 97(7): 1275–1282. doi: 10.2105/ajph.2006.091827.

Gee, G. C., Spencer, M., Chen, J., Yip, T., and Takeuchi, D. T. (2007b). The association between self-reported racial discrimination and 12-month DSM-IV mental disorders among Asian Americans nationwide. *Social Science and Medicine* 64(10): 1984–1996. doi: 10.1016/j.socscimed.2007.02.013.

Green, A. R., Carney, D. R., Pallin, D. J., Ngo, L. H., Raymond, K. L., Iezzoni, L. I., and Banaji, M. R. (2007). Implicit bias among physicians and its prediction of thrombolysis decisions for black and white patients. *Journal of General Internal Medicine* 22(9): 1231–1238. doi: 10.1007/s11606-007-0258-5.

Greene, M. P., and Blitz, L. V. (2011). The elephant is not pink: Talking about white, black, and brown to achieve excellence in clinical practice. *Clinical Social Work Journal* 40(2): 203–212. doi: 10.1007/s10615-011-0357-y.

Grier-Reed, T. L. (2010). The African American student network: Creating sanctuaries and counterspaces for coping with racial microaggressions in higher education settings. *Journal of Humanistic Counseling, Education and Development* 49(2): 181–188. doi: 10.1002/j.2161-1939.2010.tb00096.x.

Hamilton, J. (2009). Intercultural competence in medical education—essential to acquire, difficult to assess. *Medical Teacher* 31(9): 862–865. doi: 10.1080/01421590802530906.

Harrell, J. P., Hall, S., and Taliaferro, J. (2003). Physiological responses to racism and discrimination: An assessment of the evidence. *American Journal of Public Health* 93(2): 243–248. doi: 10.2105/ajph.93.2.243.

Hassed, C., de Lisle, S., Sullivan, G., and Pier, C. (2008). Enhancing the health of medical students: Outcomes of an integrated mindfulness and lifestyle program. *Advances in Health Sciences Education* 14(3): 387–398. doi: 10.1007/s10459-008-9125-3.

Hatzenbuehler, M. L., Nolen-Hoeksema, S., and Dovidio, J. (2009). How does stigma "get under the skin"? *Psychological Science* 20(10): 1282–1289. doi: 10.1111/j.1467-9280.2009.02441.x.

Herek, G. M. (2009). Hate crimes and stigma-related experiences among sexual minority adults in the United States: Prevalence estimates from a national probability sample. *Journal of Interpersonal Violence* 24(1): 54–74. doi: 10.1177/0886260508316477.

Hernández, P., Carranza, M., and Almeida, R. (2010). Mental health professionals' adaptive responses to racial microaggressions: An exploratory study. *Professional Psychology: Research and Practice* 41(3): 202–209. doi: 10.1037/a0018445.

Irving, J. A., Dobkin, P. L., and Park, J. (2009). Cultivating mindfulness in health care professionals: A review of empirical studies of mindfulness-based stress reduction (MBSR). *Complementary Therapies in Clinical Practice,* 15(2): 61–66. doi: 10.1016/j.ctcp.2009.01.002.

Koenig, H. G., Hooten, E. G., Lindsay-Calkins, E., and Meador, K. G. (2010). Spirituality in medical school curricula: Findings from a national survey. *International Journal of Psychiatry in Medicine* 40(4): 391–398. doi: 10.2190/pm.40.4.c.

Krieger, N., and Sidney, S. (1996). Racial discrimination and blood pressure: The CARDIA Study of young black and white adults. *American Journal of Public Health* 86(10): 1370–1378. doi: 10.2105/ajph.86.10.1370.

Laird, T. F., Engberg, M. E., and Hurtado, S. (2005). Modeling accentuation effects: Enrolling in a diversity course and the importance of social action engagement. *Journal of Higher Education* 76(4): 448–476. doi: 10.1353/jhe.2005.0028.

Laursen, S. L., Austin, A. E., Soto, M., and Martinez, D. (2015). ADVANCing the agenda for gender equity. *Change: Magazine of Higher Learning* 47(4): 16–24. doi: 10.1080/00091383.2015.1053767.

Lautenberger, D.M., Dandar, V.M., Raezer, C.L., Sloane, R.A. (2014). *The state of women in academic medicine: The pipeline and pathways to leadership.* Retrieved February 4, 2017, from https://www.aamc.org/members/gwims/statistics.

Lopez, L., Vranceanu, A., Cohen, A. P., Betancourt, J., and Weissman, J. S. (2008). Personal characteristics associated with resident physicians' self perceptions of preparedness to deliver cross-cultural care. *Journal of General Internal Medicine* 23(12): 1953–1958. doi: 10.1007/s11606-008-0782-y.

Mader, E. M., Rodríguez, J. E., Campbell, K. M., Smilnak, T., Bazemore, A. W., Petterson, S., and Morley, C. P. (2016). Status of underrepresented minority and female faculty at medical schools located within Historically Black Colleges and in Puerto Rico. *Medical Education Online* 21(1): 29535. doi: 10.3402/meo.v21.29535.

Mansh, M., White, W., Gee-Tong, L., Lunn, M. R., Obedin-Maliver, J., Stewart, L., et al. (2015). Sexual and gender minority identity disclosure during undergraduate medical education. *Academic Medicine* 90(5): 634–644. doi: 10.1097/acm.0000000000000657.

Mays, V. M., Cochran, S. D., and Barnes, N. W. (2007). Race, race-based discrimination, and health outcomes among African Americans. *Annual Review of Psychology* 58(1): 201–225. doi: 10.1146/annurev.psych.57.102904.190212.

Morahan, P. S., Rosen, S. E., Richman, R. C., and Gleason, K. A. (2011). The leadership continuum: A framework for organizational and individual assessment relative to the advancement of women physicians and scientists. *Journal of Women's Health* 20(3): 387–396. doi: 10.1089/jwh.2010.2055.

Nadal, K. L., Whitman, C. N., Davis, L. S., Erazo, T., and Davidoff, K. C. (2016). Microaggressions toward lesbian, gay, bisexual, transgender, queer, and genderqueer people: A review of the literature. *Journal of Sex Research* 53(4–5): 488–508. doi: 10.1080/00224499.2016.1142495.

Odom, K. L., Roberts, L. M., Johnson, R. L., and Cooper, L. A. (2007). Exploring obstacles to and opportunities for professional success among ethnic minority medical students. *Academic Medicine* 82(2): 146–153. doi: 10.1097/acm.0b013e31802d8f2c.

Orom, H., Semalulu, T., and Underwood, W. (2013). The social and learning environments experienced by underrepresented minority medical students. *Academic Medicine* 88(11): 1765–1777. doi: 10.1097/acm.0b013e3182a7a3af.

Perez, T., Hattis, P., and Barnett, K. (2007). *Health professions accreditation and diversity: A review of current standards and processes.* Battle Creek, MI: Kellogg Foundation.

Przedworski, J. M., Dovidio, J. F., Hardeman, R. R., Phelan, S. M., Burke, S. E., Ruben, M. A., et al. (2015). A comparison of the mental health and well-being of sexual minority and heterosexual first-year medical students. *Academic Medicine* 90(5): 652–659. doi: 10.1097/acm.0000000000000658.

Rosenzweig, S., Reibel, D. K., Greeson, J. M., Brainard, G. C., and Hojat, M. (2003). Mindfulness-based stress reduction lowers psychological distress in medical students. *Teaching and Learning in Medicine* 15(2): 88–92. doi: 10.1207/s15328015tlm1502_03.

Saha, S., Guiton, G., Wimmers, P. F., and Wilkerson, L. (2008). Student body racial and ethnic composition and diversity-related outcomes in U.S. medical schools. *JAMA* 300(10): 1135–1145. doi: 10.1001/jama.300.10.1135.

Salvatore, J., and Shelton, J. N. (2007). Cognitive costs of exposure to racial prejudice. *Psychological Science* 18(9): 810–815. doi: 10.1111/j.1467–9280.2007.01984.x.

Sánchez, J., Peters, L., Lee-Rey, E., Strelnick, H., Garrison, G., Zhang, K., et al. (2013). Racial and ethnic minority medical students' perceptions of and interest in careers in academic medicine. *Academic Medicine* 88(9): 1299–1307. doi: 10.1097/acm.0b013e31829f87a7.

Solorzano, D., Ceja, M., and Yosso, T. (2000). Critical race theory, racial microaggressions, and campus racial climate: The experiences of African American college students. *Journal of Negro Education* 69(1/2): 60–73.

Steele, C. M. (2011). *Whistling Vivaldi: How stereotypes affect us and what we can do.* New York: Norton.

Sue, D. W. (2010). *Microaggressions in everyday life: Race, gender, and sexual orientation.* Hoboken, NJ: Wiley.

Sue, D. W., Capodilupo, C. M., Torino, G. C., Bucceri, J. M., Holder, A. M., Nadal, K. L., and Esquilin, M. (2007). Racial microaggressions in everyday life: Implications for clinical practice. *American Psychologist* 62(4): 271–286. doi: 10.1037/0003-066x.62.4.271.

Taylor, V., and Rust, G. S. (1999). The needs of students from diverse cultures. *Academic Medicine* 74(4): 302–304. doi: 10.1097/00001888-199904000-00006.

United States Census Bureau (U.S. Census Bureau). (2016). Population estimates, July 1, 2016 (V2016). Retrieved March 2017 from https://www.census.gov/quickfacts/table/PST045216/00.

van Ryn, M., Hardeman, R., Phelan, S. M., Ph.D., D. J., Dovidio, J. F., Herrin, J., et al. (2015). Medical school experiences associated with change in implicit racial bias among 3,547 students: A medical student CHANGES study report. *Journal of General Internal Medicine* 30(12): 1748–1756. doi: 10.1007/s11606-015-3447-7.

Warnecke, E., Quinn, S., Ogden, K., Towle, N., and Nelson, M. R. (2011). A randomised controlled trial of the effects of mindfulness practice on medical student stress levels. *Medical Education* 45(4): 381–388. doi: 10.1111/j.1365-2923.2010.03877.x.

West, L. M., Donovan, R. A., and Roemer, L. (2009). Coping with racism: What works and doesn't work for black women? *Journal of Black Psychology* 36(3): 331–349. doi: 10.1177/0095798409353755.

Wong, G., Derthick, A. O., David, E., Saw, A., and Okazaki, S. (2014). The what, the why, and the how: A review of racial microaggressions research in psychology. *Race and Social Problems* 6(2): 181–200.

Yu, P. T., Parsa, P. V., Hassanein, O., Rogers, S. O., and Chang, D. C. (2013). Minorities struggle to advance in academic medicine: A 12-year review of diversity at the highest levels of America's teaching institutions. *Journal of Surgical Research* 182(2): 212–218. doi: 10.1016/j.jss.2012.06.049.

Zea, M. C., Jarama, S. L., and Bianchi, F. T. (1995). Social support and psychosocial competence: Explaining the adaptation to college of ethnically diverse students. *American Journal of Community Psychology* 23(4): 509–531. doi: 10.1007/bf02506966.

7

Courage in Medicine

JOHN MASSINI, NILA RADHAKRISHNAN, AND ERIC I. ROSENBERG[1]

Primum non tacere—First, do not be silent.

Socrates

In this chapter we discuss how learners may fear speaking up in opposition to senior members of the instructional hierarchy. We describe strategies by which institutions can develop a safe environment where learners feel comfortable advocating in the setting of ethical dilemmas.

Objectives

Describe the concept of *parrhesia* as it applies to clinical learners.
Discuss why learners may be hesitant to acknowledge ethical dilemmas.
Describe common ethical dilemmas encountered by learners.
Describe methods that medical institutions can use to instill a culture of taking courage in medicine.

Following morning "lightning" rounds (during which we had seen 20 patients in half an hour), my resident asked me to write SOAP notes in five charts. I felt uneasy because I had not actually examined these patients and wasn't sure if anybody had done a routine morn-

---

1   John Massini, M.D., University of Florida College of Medicine and Malcom Randall VA, Gainesville, FL.
Nila Radhakrishnan, M.D., University of Florida College of Medicine, Gainesville, FL.
Eric I. Rosenberg, M.D., M.S.P.H., F.A.C.P., University of Florida College of Medicine, Gainesville, FL.

ing physical exam. But the whole team was doing it and I wanted to fit in, so I complied.

Anonymous medical student (Feudtner et al. 1994)

In this chapter, we discuss how to accept the responsibility and cultivate the courage to "speak up" in ethically challenging situations that arise during medical training. Dwyer's citing of Socrates' apt maxim, *primum non tacere*, elevates the importance of speaking up to that of "first, do no harm" (1994). The "hidden curriculum," consisting of behaviors role-modeled by clinicians, can lead learners to overlook and normalize ethically concerning behavior (Hafferty 1998). A recent study reports that 64 percent of learners personally observed at least one instance of unprofessional behavior during the four years of medical school (Hendelman and Byszewski 2014). Arrogance on the part of attending physicians, nurses, or fellow students was the example most frequently reported by learners. Closely following arrogance were impairment, breaches of confidentiality, unconscientious behavior, cultural/religious insensitivity, and abuse of power (Hendelman and Byszewski 2014). Feudtner et al. report student dissatisfaction with their own actions, with 67 percent feeling bad or remorseful about something they had done (Feudtner et al. 1994).

Health professionals have a fiduciary responsibility to pursue a course of action that is always in the patient's best interest. For learners, this obligation may lead to conflict with more senior clinicians when learners perceive that they better understand or advocate for the patient's perspective. Additional tension can arise because, while attending physicians are licensed, credentialed, and financially compensated by the patient to provide care, learners are trained to develop and exercise progressive autonomy. Learners often rapidly and more readily empathize with a patient's perspective and care preferences (Feudtner et al. 1994). However, learners can feel tremendous pressure to defer to authority and to those with more knowledge and experience. They may fear that speaking up in opposition to senior members on the team could jeopardize their grades, letters of recommendation, and the trajectory of their postgraduate training careers (Feudtner et al. 1994). Learners' goals of studying medicine, being "good team players," and caring for patients are all admirable. Yet conflicts between these objectives contribute to frequently observed scenarios that are ethically complex and challenging.

Learners experience intense emotions during their training, accompanied by high stress levels. They see patients receive cancer diagnoses and participate in end-of-life discussions. Perhaps because they have additional time available to spend at the bedside and are first call in the chain of command, learners often spend the most time with a patient and hear about patients' frustrations firsthand. Many learners feel unqualified due to their lack of experience, yet may feel pressure to perform to achieve good evaluations (Henning et al. 1998). Additionally, with clinical work and studying taking up so much time, many learners find less time to spend relaxing with friends and family or on leisure activities (Lee and Graham 2001). Because of these and other risk factors, one study found that 14.3 percent of medical students experienced moderate to severe depression and 4.4 percent reported suicidal ideation during medical school (Schwenk et al. 2010). During stressful periods like this, humor is a coping mechanism that can reduce perceived stress (Abel 2002). However, when humor is derogatory toward patients, it may result in learner cynicism and unprofessional behavior (Wear et al. 2009).

Ethics courses have long been present in medical school curricula to discuss these issues, but such courses are insufficient to create an ethical culture (Feudtner et al. 1994). We will discuss ways medical institutions have worked to instill a culture of professionalism that persists beyond preclinical activities.

Conceptual Framework: *Parrhesia* (Fearless Speech)

Foucault gave six lectures in 1983 devoted to the concept of *parrhesia*, or "frankness in speaking the truth" (Foucault and Pearson 2001). There are several layers of nuance to the term that go deeper than just the ability to say what one wants. *Parrhesia* is a form of criticism in which the person speaking, or *parrhesiastes*, is in a position of inferiority to the person being criticized. Thus, voicing a concern carries risk to the speaker. Not just anyone had the status to speak with *parrhesia*. In the original Greek concept, as Foucault describes, only citizens of Athens were worthy of this right. In order for *parrhesia* to apply to speech, there must be a duty on the part of the *parrhesiastes* to speak up (2001).

Papadimos and Murray (2008) introduce the concept of *parrhesia* as it relates to medical learners. Medical schools select future physicians to study clinical medicine based on their demonstrated honesty, integrity, intellect, and discipline. These same qualities give clinical learners the right and responsibility of *parrhesia*. The clinical learner has an elevated status compared with those who have not received medical education, but ranks lower than the attending physician. Potential risks for clinical learners who criticize a senior team member include lower evaluations, ostracization, and lack of teaching. However, if learners witness behavior jeopardizing patient safety or the fiduciary relationship between physicians and patients, they have a duty to speak up despite the personal risk. Clinical teachers can allow the practice of *parrhesia* by providing an environment where free speech is encouraged.

Categorization of Clinical Scenarios That Compel *Parrhesia*

The duty of *parrhesia* in medical learners is fundamentally linked to professionalism. However, there are many ways to describe professionalism and no single set of universally accepted criteria that define it. The American Board of Internal Medicine defines the "Elements of Professionalism" to be altruism, accountability, excellence, duty, honor, integrity, and respect for others (Robins et al. 2002). Contrasting elements include abuse of power, breach of confidentiality, bias, sexual harassment, arrogance, greed, misrepresentation, impairment, lack of conscientiousness, conflicts of interest, and conflicts of conscience (Hendelman and Byszewski 2014).

Several authors followed the spirit of the Ritchie/Spencer five-step process for qualitative data analysis (Ritchie and Spencer 2002) by collecting student vignettes, consulting references such as ethics textbooks or curricula, formulating tentative initial categories of professionalism violations, mapping the vignettes to the categories, then adjusting the categories to more effectively characterize the types of lapses students were witnessing (Caldicott and Faber-Langendoen 2005; Christakis and Feudtner 1993; Feudtner et al. 1994; Monrouxe et al. 2011; Myers and Herb 2013; Rees et al. 2013; Rosenbaum et al. 2004; Satterwhite et al. 1998).

After comparing examples and categories of relevant clinical scenarios in the literature, we have identified a list of common ethical dilemmas, outlined below, that compel learners to respond with *parrhesia* (Caldicott and Faber-Langendoen 2005; Christakis and Feudtner 1993; Fard et al. 2010; Feudtner et al. 1994; Hendelman and Byszewski 2014; Monrouxe et al. 2011; Myers and Herb 2013; Rees et al. 2013; Robins et al. 2002; Rosenbaum et al. 2004; Satterwhite et al. 1998).

Common Ethical Dilemmas That Compel *Parrhesia*

Witnessing unethical behavior by other team members

Learners in medical training programs have reported witnessing many types of unethical behavior. These reports include seeing senior teammates chemically restrain nonconsenting capacitated patients, watching residents perform unnecessary forceps deliveries "for practice," and uncomfortably holding a patient's hand as a resident performed a biopsy of a vulvar lesion against her expressed wishes (Christakis and Feudtner 1993). Sometimes senior members on the team intimidate and humiliate lower ranked members of the team in order to deny and deflect blame. Over time, witnessing repeated uncorrected breaches in professionalism can normalize the behavior. This pattern can affect learners' own attitudes and may undermine formal professionalism training (D'Eon et al. 2007; Pololi and Price 2000).

Learners observe clinical preceptors talking to patients and families and explaining clinical care. An ethical dilemma arises if they hear a patient being given deceptive or false information. Below is a vignette from a learner caring for a patient in an emergency department (ED) who had been transferred from another facility to further evaluate an abnormal head CT. The student and ED physician reviewed the images, but did not speak with a radiologist.

> I was surprised to hear the attending tell the family, "We've had our expert neuro-radiologists, who specialize in CT scans of the head, review the films." . . . I had been in possession of the CD the entire time. Why did this attending lie to this family? Would they feel even more assured knowing a neuro-radiologist had read the film? Would they have not trusted an emergency room physician's opinion? Would they feel better when they got their bill for the helicopter? . . . I still do not fully understand this physician's motivation for lying. I debated whether I should bring up the issue with the physician but could not think of a good way to broach the subject. (Santen and Hemphill 2011, p. 291)

In one study by Caldicott and Faber-Langendoen (2005), deliberately lying to or deceiving the patient was the most commonly described ethical lapse out of 40 primary issues identified. In some instances, learners saw deliberate lies in a positive light when they that felt the deception advocated for the patient. An example is the doctor who writes for a child's prescription in the mother's name because the mother has insurance and the child does not (Caldicott and Faber-Langendoen 2005). The doctor acts out of a desire to do well, but learners may not yet grasp the risks to individual and professional credibility caused by well-intentioned acts of dishonesty.

Another category of ethical lapses related to deceiving a patient is directing a learner to perform an invasive procedure if she is not comfortable performing it, the procedure is being done against the patient's will, or the patient gave express instructions to have an attending physician perform the procedure (Caldicott and Faber-Langendoen 2005; Christakis and Feudtner 1993). In the vignette below, a learner describes a scenario in which a teacher wants to demonstrate an exam. The learner, however, notes that the patient did not have an opportunity to consent.

[I] had gained consent to watch a vaginal examination of an elderly lady. I was watching and consultant said: "[Name], put on a glove." Once I had done [so] he instructed me to feel the ring he had inserted into the vaginal entrance. After I looked at the patient and started to ask for consent, he cut me off saying, "You don't mind if he feels do you, he's just a doctor in training and needs to know how it feels." [This was stated as] very much a statement rather than [a] question. (Rees et al. 2013, p. 86)

The gynecologic examination is a crucial opportunity to demonstrate respect and professionalism. The attending physician could have taught the student appropriate language to use when describing the procedure and could have discussed pelvic examination by the learner while the patient was still dressed. It is degrading for patient and learner when the attending physician uses coercion to enable a learner to perform the examination. This behavior teaches the learner that consent is not important. Practicing *parrhesia* in this case would entail the learner having the courage to ask the patient for consent and later discuss with the physician the importance of consent. It is the responsibility of medical educators to create an environment within the clinical setting which encourages the practice of *parrhesia*.

Conflict between being a team player and honoring duty to patients

As students, we become overly concerned with grades. Students should speak up when it concerns the patient. If we do not, we are as guilty as the individuals who violate patients' values.

Anonymous medical student (Caldicott and Faber-Langendoen 2005, p. 870)

Several papers describe the learners' fear of speaking up to instructors (Caldicott and Faber-Langendoen 2005; Feudtner et al. 1994). In the clinical setting, students learn from nurses, interns, senior residents, and the attending. Since learners have a limited knowledge base and less experience than their instructors, they may feel hesitant to confront a senior member of the team about a decision that does not feel ethical. In one scenario, a student was concerned about an abnormal lab test result on the planned day of discharge. The resident told the student not to bring it up or document it because the "super-cautious" attending would have kept the patient in the hospital (Feudtner et al. 1994). In some settings, learners may remain silent not out of fear but because they feel they are "bothering" the instructor with clinical issues that they "should" be able to solve themselves. For example, learners have described neglecting to report a patient's symptoms to the instructor so as not to "bother" the instructor (Feudtner et al. 1994). Learners want to be "team players" and, when told to do so, may perform tasks without adequate supervision. Some instructors have asked students to obtain informed consent, a nondelegable physician responsibility (Christakis and Feudtner 1993). Assigning this task to a student without physician involvement could likely mean the patient is not fully informed about the procedure and could receive incorrect information in response to their questions.

In hospital medicine, although the attending physician is thought of as the senior member of a team of learners, it is also notable that the learners themselves make up a subteam. Students generally spend more time with the interns and residents than they do with the attending physician. Students feel pressure not to make the interns and residents appear incompetent or unprepared in front of the attending (Feudtner et al. 1994). However, unwillingness to speak against the team can act as a barrier to communicating important information to the attending. For example, a learner may hesitate to bring up clinical issues to the attending or senior physician for fear that this would highlight issues that the interns or residents failed to solve. Pressure to fit in with the team can also tempt a learner to go along with questionable practices in order to help things run smoothly, as in the vignette that starts this chapter.

Learners can feel powerless in their low position in the chain of command. They may feel that speaking up is pointless, because their concerns could be easily dismissed by more senior members of the team. Learners may also feel that speaking up would place them at odds with the rest of the team for the remainder of the rotation. Thus, the practice of *parrhesia* will probably not occur easily in a setting where it is not encouraged. In such settings, even if a learner approaches the teacher with respect, *parrhesia* is most frequently received as a challenge to the status quo and the attending's judgment (Wear et al. 2011). Learners often use this risk of offending others as a justification for allowing breaches in professionalism, even if the breach may compromise patient safety. Sometimes learners may speak up but find that their concerns are shrugged off without serious consideration. When students' concerns about exam findings are not investigated, or when their questions are trivialized or dealt with curtly, this dismissal may discourage them from speaking up and pointing out something important later (Dwyer 1994). In the past 20 years, the movement for a quality and patient safety culture has helped create an environment where anyone caring for a patient has the right and responsibility to speak up about patient safety issues. Medical educators and clinical educators face the similar challenge of creating an environment that encourages *parrhesia*.

Witnessing lack of respect for others

Since learners care for fewer patients than other team members, they have more time to spend getting to know patients personally. In one study, 92 percent of students believed "they knew their patients as people better than other team members" (Feudtner et al. 1994, p. 673). This familiarity with patients is a positive aspect of their training, but it heightens the conflict felt by the student if team members disrespect the patient's wishes or say something inappropriate. Students can also feel torn if they are instructed to withhold information from a patient (Feudtner et al. 1994).

Gallows humor and derogatory humor

Humor has many positive effects: it can strengthen relationships, relieve anxiety, release anger in a socially acceptable way, avoid/deny painful feelings, and facilitate learning (Robinson 1991). Gallows humor "treats serious, frightening, or painful subject matter in a light or satirical way" (Watson 2011, p. 38). Derogatory humor, however, takes matters a step further and is more mean-spirited. One physician characterized the distinction between gallows humor and derogatory humor as the difference between "whistling as you go through the graveyard" and "kicking over the gravestones" (Wear et al. 2009, p. 39). However, the line can be blurry. Although physicians may employ gallows humor to deal with difficult situations, build relationships with colleagues, or communicate the truth more rapidly than ordinary etiquette would allow, it can confuse learners by depersonalizing and disrespecting patients (Watson 2011). A tired resident at the end of a stressful shift with a severely ill patient may that say their patient was "trying to die" or that the patient is "circling the drain." Teammates may give each other high fives after discharging a particularly unpleasant patient (Sobel 2006). An intern may chuckle about a "code brown" when he examined a patient who suffered an uncontrollable bowel movement. This behavior may not feel inappropriate in the confines of the team room, but would be hurtful if said in front of and understood by the patient. Medical learners who have not normalized this type of humor can start to experience burnout from the "negative energy" emanating from a team with a culture of derogatory humor (Wear et al. 2009). Even if the patient never hears the actual joking in a doctors' workroom, it can influence the doctor-patient relationship by gradually changing the way a doctor-in-training views the patient (McCrary and Christensen 1993). Slang terms may be a form of derogatory humor. For example, referring to a patient as a "rock" because she has had a prolonged hospitalization and is unable to return home due to debility, comorbidity, or limited financial means is inappropriate, may indicate resentment, and generates a perception of the patient as a burden to the physician. Dr. Stephen Bergman's 1978 novel *The House of God* is familiar to most medical students and residents as an infamous fictional description of the stresses of residency training in internal medicine and the role of dark humor as a coping mechanism. Although the book is a satirical and sobering look at the need for doctors to maintain their empathy and change the nature of 1970s medical education, today's learners are still likely at times to hear patients described with phrases attributed to the novel, such as "train wrecks." Learners may adopt this new vocabulary out of a desire to fit in with the accepted culture, but also may feel uncomfortable and disillusioned. As with the other lapses in professionalism, students may be concerned that speaking out against this type of humor could turn team members against them.

In 2015, an anesthesiologist was recorded making fun of a sedated patient during his colonoscopy, resulting in extensive publicity.

> When a medical assistant noted the man had a rash, the anesthesiologist warned her not to touch it, saying she might get "some syphilis on [her] arm or something," then added, "It's probably tuberculosis in the penis, so you'll be alright." (Jackman 2015)

Unprofessional behavior such as using derogatory humor shatters trust in the medical profession. We shouldn't avoid disrespectful language toward patients because of fear that we may be recorded; we should respect patients because it is our duty. Patients place their trust in us by divulging personal information they share with no one else. They place their trust in us by consenting to anesthesia that renders them helpless. We owe it to them to demonstrate that we are worthy of that trust. Clinical learners need the courage to question humor that ridicules or humiliates patients and diminishes the professionalism of the physician. Similarly, clinical teachers have a responsibility to model professional behavior and create an environment where learners are encouraged to speak freely, with *parrhesia*.

Lack of justice

Justice and discrimination comprise another category of lapses in professionalism between doctors and patients (Caldicott and Faber-Langendoen 2005). This category includes cases where vulnerable patients receive discriminatory treatment based on socioeconomic status, personal characteristics, or self-induced illness—for example, making derogatory comments about a patient who is a prisoner or treating her with less compassion or diligence (Caldicott and Faber-Langendoen 2005). One student saw a surgeon perform staple closure of an incision differently on a cerebral palsy patient compared to an attractive young girl (Caldicott and Faber-Langendoen 2005). Was scarring irrelevant to the patient with cerebral palsy? The learner in these situations has the opportunity and the duty to speak with *parrhesia* on behalf of the cerebral palsy patient.

Arrogance

Arrogance can tear apart a team and act as a wedge between the doctor and patient. Arrogant behavior can happen between doctors and patients, doctors and nurses or ancillary staff, senior members of the medical team and subordinates, or different consulting teams taking care of the same patient. As Berger (2002) notes, "It behooves each of us as physicians to remember that we are but instruments of healing and not its source" (Berger 2002, p. 147). Learners have a duty to speak up for patient respect with *parrhesia* and, if arrogance blinds a senior team member to important details in the case or undermines the doctor-patient relationship, to advocate for the patient's perspective.

Impairment

Physician and learner impairment due to substance abuse, mental illness, or other illness (for example, severely uncontrolled, newly presenting diabetes) can be disruptive on many levels. Patient safety, teaching, and learning can be compromised. Physician impairment due to substance abuse can go unnoticed for a long time, particularly since work is one of the later aspects of life to be affected. It may present as unreliability, lack of interest, or erratic behavior. In rare, tragic situations, residents have over-dosed in call rooms (Krizek 2004). Rehabilitation of impaired physicians is often effective, and it is critical to support these people and get them the help they need (Yellowlees et al. 2014). A learner may feel uncomfortable talking with or reporting a colleague or team member whom they suspect could have a problem with impairment. However, identifying and addressing impairment is our duty to our patients and colleagues. Summoning the courage to speak with *parrhesia* in these situations is the only way to keep our patients safe and to provide a path to healing the impaired physician or learner.

Solutions

Conflicts between the goals of caring for the patient, being a good team-mate, and learning how to be a physician can cause our learners to stumble into a dark wood. Although the right path is unmistakable in second-year ethics lectures, the third- or fourth-year student on the wards can have difficulty discerning it without a guide. Professionalism, like quality, is not a finish line that can be crossed. It is a process of identifying problems and working consistently to improve. Just as systems and institutional culture can make medical errors more or less likely, external factors can encourage physicians to speak up about professionalism or to brush problems under the rug.

The first step in educating learners about professionalism is to address the right problems at the right time. Learners are not yet physicians, and the ethical issues they encounter are not identical to those in practice (Feudtner et al. 1994). Therefore, an appropriately targeted ethics curriculum should include discussion of vignettes that learners experience during their clinical years and "attempt to provide timely and practical guidance" (Feudtner et al. 1994, p. 678). For example, rather than only including dramatic vignettes from high-profile national cases, ethical courses should discuss cases that highlight conflicts between patient interest and being a team player. The continuing nature of professional development makes it important to have ongoing ethics discussions throughout learners' third and fourth year of training. The Internal Medicine clerkship at the University of Florida tasks students with a written reflection on a positive or negative incident that strongly affected them (Fischer et al. 2008). Learners meet as a group with a clinical faculty moderator and discuss each story. At the end of each year, the internal medicine clerkship director reads some anonymized examples of the positive and negative highlights of these sessions to the entire internal medicine department at grand rounds. This makes it harder for our department to slide into denial, thinking that ethical lapses only happen "somewhere else." These stories can inspire everyone to make a positive difference.

Another step is to designate a point person for learners to discuss ethical issues. This person could be the leader of an office of professionalism or a designated physician or ethicist within the department.

Thirdly, institutions can demonstrate a commitment to professionalism by developing a code of conduct. This code can be developed at various levels—at the preclinical student level, with reaffirmation at the clinical student level; at the resident/fellow level; and at the faculty level. For example, at the University of Florida College of Medicine, each student class writes their own personalized version of the Hippocratic Oath and pledges to uphold it at the White Coat Ceremony.

Institutions can also encourage professionalism by recognizing people who act professionally in challenging situations. This recognition identifies good role models and demonstrates that the institution values professionalism. Some programs hold workshops on professionalism that emphasize role modeling (Hendelman and Byszewski 2014). The Gold Humanism Society is an example of an organization that recognizes good role models and encourages high professionalism standards.

Another step in professionalism education is asking learners to evaluate members of their team on professionalism. Lapses in a physician's professionalism should result in remediation, which could lead to their removal from the learners' circle of influence. If a habitual offender never suffers any consequences, the institution is sending a message of tacit approval of the unprofessional behavior.

> Courage should not be necessary for any health care professional
> to ask a question or make a suggestion regarding a patient's care.
> (Hamric et al. 2015, p. 39)

A culture of safety, professionalism, and respect is essential to moving forward as a professional institution. Just as with medical errors, ignoring the problem perpetuates it. Departments need to make it clear from the top down that students will not be penalized for raising concerns or suggestions for how professionalism can be improved. Within a team, an attending can emphasize that calling him or her about serious concerns is acceptable and encouraged rather than an annoying inconvenience that will result in a bad evaluation. The attending should set clear expectations of residents and interns regarding professionalism and student interaction. He or she could name and recognize the pressures that students feel in this role and provide some important examples of when a student spoke up to the benefit of the patient. By ensuring nonretaliation at the beginning and prioritizing patient well-being, the attending can lower barriers to speaking up on behalf of patients and can encourage a culture of *parrhesia*.

Final Thoughts

These interventions help to encourage a culture of professionalism and respect, but they are only as good as the people on the ground. Unprofessionalism can grow into a tangled jungle for learners if no one is tending the garden. With regular maintenance and attention, we can give students the courage to do the right thing and to be a light to those around them.

Returning to the scenario at the start of the chapter, if the training program encouraged a culture of *parrhesia* through role modeling by residents themselves, it is possible that all trainees would have greater awareness of the importance of professionalism. Increased awareness by residents is critical, as they serve as role models for others and steer the culture of the team. Medical schools should also develop programs where they train students to be able to take the right moral steps when in difficult situations.

Questions for Future Research

Determine whether professionalism interventions in medical school result in lasting changes in attitudes.

Describe the impact of action research involving compiling and distributing acts of *parrhesia* at an institution.

Describe the impact of training residents to explicitly role-model professional behavior.

Study the impact Gold Humanism awardees or institutionally recognized individuals can have on the culture at an institution, clinical service, or team.

References

Abel, M. H. (2002). Humor, stress, and coping strategies. *Humor—International Journal of Humor Research* 15(4): 365–381. doi: 10.1515/humr.15.4.365.

Berger, A. S. (2002). Arrogance among physicians. *Academic Medicine* 77(2): 145–147. doi: 10.1097/00001888-200202000-00010.

Caldicott, C. V., and Faber-Langendoen, K. (2005). Deception, discrimination, and fear of reprisal: Lessons in ethics from third-year medical students. *Academic Medicine* 80(9): 866–873. doi: 10.1097/00001888-200509000-00018.

Christakis, D. A., and Feudtner, C. (1993). Ethics in a short white coat. *Academic Medicine* 68(4): 249–254. doi: 10.1097/00001888-199304000-00003.

D'Eon, M., Lear, N., Turner, M., and Jones, C. (2007). Perils of the hidden curriculum revisited. *Medical Teacher* 29(4): 295–296. doi: 10.1080/01421590701291485.

Dwyer, J. (1994). Primum non tacere: An ethics of speaking up. *Hastings Center Report* 24(1): 13. doi: 10.2307/3562380.

Fard, N. N., Asghari, F., and Mirzazadeh, A. (2010). Ethical issues confronted by medical students during clinical rotations. *Medical Education* 44(7): 723–730. doi: 10.1111/j.1365-2923.2010.03671.x.

Feudtner, C., Christakis, D. A., and Christakis, N. A. (1994). Do clinical clerks suffer ethical erosion? Students' perceptions of their ethical environment and personal development. *Academic Medicine* 69(8): 670–679. doi: 10.1097/00001888-199408000-00017.

Fischer, M. A., Harrell, H. E., Haley, H., Cifu, A. S., Alper, E., Johnson, K. M., and Hatem, D. (2008). Between two worlds: A multi-institutional qualitative analysis of students' reflections on joining the medical profession. *Journal of General Internal Medicine* 23(7): 958–963. doi: 10.1007/s11606-008-0508-1.

Foucault, M., and Pearson, J. (2001). *Fearless speech*. Los Angeles, CA: Semiotext(e).

Hafferty, F. W. (1998). Beyond curriculum reform: Confronting medicine's hidden curriculum. *Academic Medicine* 73(4): 403–407. doi: 10.1097/00001888-199804000-00013.

Hamric, A. B., Arras, J. D., and Mohrmann, M. E. (2015). Must we be courageous? *Hastings Center Report* 45(3): 33–40. doi: 10.1002/hast.449.

Hendelman, W., and Byszewski, A. (2014). Formation of medical student professional identity: Categorizing lapses of professionalism, and the learning environment. *BMC Medical Education* 14(139). doi: 10.1186/1472-6920-14-139.

Henning, K., Ey, S., and Shaw, D. (1998). Perfectionism, the impostor phenomenon and psychological adjustment in medical, dental, nursing and pharmacy students. *Medical Education* 32(5): 456–464. doi: 10.1046/j.1365-2923.1998.00234.x.

Jackman, T. (2015, June 23) Anesthesiologist trashes sedated patient—and it ends up costing her. *Washington Post*. Retrieved from https://www.washingtonpost.com/local/anesthesiologist-trashes-sedated-patient-jury-orders-her-to-pay-500000/2015/06/23/cae05c00-18f3-11e5-ab92-c75ae6ab94b5_story.html?utm_term=.1c231c6df4fb.

Krizek, T. J. (2004). The impaired surgical resident. *Surgical Clinics of North America* 84(6): 1587–1604. doi: 10.1016/j.suc.2004.06.016.

Lee, J., and Graham, A. V. (2001). Students' perception of medical school stress and their evaluation of a wellness elective. *Medical Education* 35(7): 652–659. doi: 10.1046/j.1365-2923.2001.00956.x.

McCrary, S., and Christensen, R. C. (1993). Slang "on board." A moral analysis of medical jargon. *Archives of Family Medicine* 2(1): 101–105. doi: 10.1001/archfami.2.1.101.

Monrouxe, L. V., Rees, C. E., and Hu, W. (2011). Differences in medical students' explicit discourses of professionalism: Acting, representing, becoming. *Medical Education* 45(6): 585–602. doi: 10.1111/j.1365-2923.2010.03878.x.

Myers, M. F., and Herb, A. (2013). Ethical dilemmas in clerkship rotations. *Academic Medicine* 88(11): 1609–1611. doi: 10.1097/acm.0b013e3182a7f919.

Papadimos, T. J., and Murray, S. J. (2008). Foucault's "fearless speech" and the transformation and mentoring of medical students. *Philosophy, Ethics, and Humanities in Medicine* 3(1): 12. doi: 10.1186/1747-5341-3-12.

Pololi, L., and Price, J. (2000). Validation and use of an instrument to measure the learning environment as perceived by medical students. *Teaching and Learning in Medicine* 12(4): 201–207. doi: 10.1207/s15328015tlm1204_7.

Rees, C. E., Monrouxe, L. V., and Mcdonald, L. A. (2013). Narrative, emotion and action: Analysing "most memorable" professionalism dilemmas. *Medical Education* 47(1): 80–96. doi: 10.1111/j.1365-2923.2012.04302.x.

Ritchie, J., and Spencer, L. (2002). Qualitative data analysis for applied policy research. In A. M. Huberman and M. B. Biles (eds.), *The qualitative researcher's companion* (pp. 305–329). doi: 10.4135/9781412986274.n12.

Robins, L. S., Braddock, C. H., and Fryer-Edwards, K. A. (2002). Using the American Board of Internal Medicine's "Elements of Professionalism" for undergraduate ethics education. *Academic Medicine* 77(6): 523–531. doi: 10.1097/00001888-200206000-00008.

Robinson, V. M. (1991). *Humor and the health professions: The therapeutic use of humor in health care.* Thorofare, NJ: Slack.

Rosenbaum, J. R., Bradley, E. H., Holmboe, E. S., Farrell, M. H., and Krumholz, H. M. (2004). Sources of ethical conflict in medical housestaff training: A qualitative study. *American Journal of Medicine* 116(6): 402–407. doi: 10.1016/j.amjmed.2003.09.044.

Santen, S. A., and Hemphill, R. R. (2011). A window on professionalism in the emergency department through medical student narratives. *Annals of Emergency Medicine* 58(3): 288–294. doi: 10.1016/j.annemergmed.2011.04.001.

Satterwhite, W. M., 3rd, Satterwhite, R. C., and Enarson, C. E. (1998). Medical students' perceptions of unethical conduct at one medical school. *Academic Medicine* 73(5): 529–531. doi: 10.1097/00001888-199805000-00021.

Schwenk, T. L., Davis, L., and Wimsatt, L. A. (2010). Depression, stigma, and suicidal ideation in medical students. *JAMA* 304(11): 1181–1190. doi: 10.1001/jama.2010.1300.

Sobel, R. K. (2006). Does Laughter Make Good Medicine? *New England Journal of Medicine* 354(11): 1114–1115. doi: 10.1056/nejmp058089.

Watson, K. (2011). Gallows humor in medicine. *Hastings Center Report* 41(5): 37–45. doi: 10.1002/j.1552-146x.2011.tb00139.x.

Wear, D., Zarconi, J., and Dhillon, N. (2011). Teaching fearlessness: A manifesto. *Education for Health* (Abingdon, England) 24(3): 668.

Wear, D., Aultman, J. M., Zarconi, J., and Varley, J. D. (2009). Derogatory and cynical humour directed towards patients: Views of residents and attending doctors. *Medical Education* 43(1): 34–41. doi: 10.1111/j.1365-2923.2008.03171.x.

Yellowlees, P. M., Campbell, M. D., Rose, J. S., Parish, M. B., Ferrer, D., Scher, L. M., . . . Dupont, R. L. (2014). Psychiatrists with substance use disorders: Positive treatment outcomes from physician health programs. *Psychiatric Services* 65(12): 1492–1495. doi: 10.1176/appi.ps.201300472.

8

The Secret in the Care of the Learner

YING NAGOSHI, PAULETTE HAHN, AND ALMA LITTLES[1]

Docendo discitur—One learns by teaching.

Seneca the Younger(?)

In this chapter, we review the literature on "pimping"[2] and mistreatment. We contrast pimping with the Socratic method of teaching and provide tips for educators to ensure a learning environment where all participants feel unthreatened, particularly by questions posed by educators.

Objectives

Describe factors that contribute to student mistreatment.

Discuss the distinction between pimping and the Socratic method as pedagogical methods.

Describe how questioning can be used by educators as a positive educational method.

Josh is a third-year medical student on his first clinical clerkship in pediatrics. On the first day of the clerkship, his attending, Dr. Jones, asks him and his fellow student several questions related to a patient. While Josh is unable to answer any of the questions, his peer is able to answer most. As the clerkship progresses, he dreads going in daily and feels increasingly anxious during rounds. He feels embarrassed, demoralized, and worthless.

---

1 Ying Nagoshi, M.D., Ph.D., University of Florida College of Medicine, Gainesville, FL.
  Paulette Hahn, M.D., M.S., University of Florida College of Medicine, Gainesville, FL.
  Alma Littles, M.D., Florida State University College of Medicine, Tallahassee, FL.
2 "When a teacher singles out one learner to ask a series of questions, sometimes with the intent to humiliate" (Scott et al. 2015).

He is worried that he will get poor evaluations and begins to question his choice of medicine as a profession.

The Struggling Learner

Research has noted several inadvertent negative effects of the medical education curriculum on students, including increased risk of depression, anxiety, and burnout (Dyrbye et al. 2006). Contributing factors include financial concerns; exposure to the "hidden curriculum of cynicism" (Dyrbye et al. 2006, p. 354); the workload for trainees, with resultant sleep deprivation and a loss of empathy; and continuous exposure to suffering (Dyrbye et al. 2006). Additionally, studies have identified profiles of students entering medical school who may be at risk for psychological distress and poor academic performance: high-risk students who lack good study skills, have poor organizational skills and knowledge base, are immature, have little or no insight, and who start medical school with an ongoing mental health problem or a personal crisis (Hays et al. 2011). A study from the United Kingdom found that 10–15 percent of the annual student intake would be identified as "strugglers" during medical school (Yates and James 2006, p. 1009). Yates and James (2006) also note that failing three or more examinations per year, suffering from health and social difficulties, failing to complete Hepatitis B vaccination on time, and eliciting remarks about a poor attitude are factors that can identify potential "strugglers." Hinson et al. (2011) also note that poor attendance or unexplained absenteeism during rotations or clinical placements is a good "proxy marker" of poor student performance (p. 33). For struggling residents and trainees, Borkett-Jones and Morris (2010) describe early warning signs, including: lateness, not answering pages, poor productivity, bursts of temper, poor tolerance of ambiguity, rejection of constructive criticism, and disillusionment with medicine. Medical schools and training programs must take proactive steps to identify learners who may be struggling academically or who have risk factors for distress and must develop support systems. For medical students, academic support strategies include study skills sessions, practice exams, individually tailored assessments and feedback, pre- and postclerkship briefings, personal professional development sessions, and academic performance appraisals (Vogan et al. 2014). For residents, educators can use workplace-based assessments, such as multisource feedback, clinical evaluation exercises like mini-CEX, and direct observation diagnostically to identify areas of concerns (Borkett-Jones and Morris 2010). Additionally, it is essential that medical schools offer a support system, which is readily accessible and consists of academic staff and mentors as well as mental health counselors, and administrative, pastoral, and other support staff trained to help students and trainees (Vogan et al. 2014).

Mistreatment of Learners

While identifying learners who are struggling is important, it is also essential to control factors in the learning environment that can result in distress, such as mistreatment and harassment of learners. Medical students in the United States report high levels of belittlement and harassment. On the Association of American Medical Colleges (AAMC) Medical School Graduation Questionnaire, 42 percent of students report at least one episode of being publicly embarrassed (AAMC 2016). Sources of public humiliation include preclerkship faculty, clerkship faculty in the classroom or in the clinical setting, residents/interns, nurses, administrators, other institution employees, and other students (AAMC 2016). The highest percentages of students reported being humiliated by clerkship faculty (12.9 percent), residents/interns (9.4 percent), and nurses (3.7 percent) (AAMC 2016). Studies have shown that this perceived mistreatment positively correlates with binge drinking, depression, anxiety, and suicidal ideation and attempts; it also results in less satisfaction with life, lower levels of confidence, and low professional satisfaction (Dyrbye et al. 2006; Frank et al. 2006; Wolf et al. 1998).

Some studies have described teaching by humiliation as a form of mistreatment. A survey of Australian medical students reported that 74 percent of students had experienced teaching by humiliation and up to 83 percent had witnessed this during clinical rotations (Scott et al. 2015). Most of the humiliating and intimidating behaviors students experienced were subtle rather than overt but included an aggressive style of questioning. Notably, however, 40 percent of the students who experienced intimidating questioning considered it useful for learning (Scott et al. 2015).

Pimping

While the *Merriam-Webster Dictionary* (*Merriam-Webster OnLine* n.d.) defines the word "pimping" as "petty, insignificant," pimping is also known as teaching by humiliation (Scott et al. 2015). Pimping is a colloquial term that strongly connotes questioning that may be abusive, intimidating, and humiliating, serving to promote the maintenance of a power hierarchy between teacher and learner, or even between learners (Reifler 2015). However, some see pimping as a valuable form of Socratic teaching (McCarthy and McEvoy 2015). Given the increasing interest in

---

Textbox 4. "Through the student's eyes: On pimping"

Umm . . .
I don't know.
Hmm . . . No, I don't know.
Don't know.

little stabbing hints . . .
. . . flop sweat.
Feeling their eyes boring into the back of my skull,
My ignorance bolstering their also battered egos.

I don't know.
The indignity. Four years my junior but R1 to my cc3.
OK, my turn:
How old was Mendelssohn when he composed *A Midsummer Night's Dream*?
What was Harpo's real name?
List for me the signs of an Auspicious Budda?
What's my favorite color?

"You're lucky you make me laugh, Libman.
Otherwise,
you'd be
worthless."

Mark Libman (Libman 2002)
Virtual Mentor, courtesy of AMA.
© 2002 American Medical Association.
All Rights Reserved.

learner resilience and in fostering humanism in medical education, it is important to understand how to provide an effective learning environment, promoting the questioning of learners as a time-honored teaching method, rather than teaching by humiliation. The Liaison Committee on Medical Education (LCME), the body that accredits medical education programs in the United States, has 12 accreditation standards. Standard 3, titled "Academic and Learning Environments," reads as follows:

> A medical school ensures that its medical education program occurs in professional, respectful, and intellectually stimulating academic and clinical environments, recognizes the benefits of diversity, and promotes students' attainment of competencies required of future physicians. (LCME 2017, p. 4)

Several pertinent elements within that standard are worth noting. Implicit in this standard is the expectation that students will be intellectually challenged, but in a manner that encourages learning as opposed to one that elicits embarrassment or causes humiliation. We describe the standards that are particularly relevant to this chapter. Element 3.2 regarding a "Community of Scholars/Research Opportunities" states:

> A medical education program is conducted in an environment that fosters the intellectual challenge and spirit of inquiry appropriate to a community of scholars and provides sufficient opportunities, encouragement, and support for medical student participation in the research and other scholarly activities of its faculty. (LCME 2017, p. 4)

Element 3.5 within that same standard, titled "Learning Environment/ Professionalism," goes on to state:

> A medical school ensures that the learning environment of its medical education program is conducive to the ongoing development of explicit and appropriate professional behaviors in its medical students, faculty, and staff at all locations and is one in which all individuals are treated with respect. (LCME 2017, p. 4)

Element 3.6 directly discusses "Student Mistreatment":

> A medical education program defines and publicizes its code of professional conduct for the relationships between medical students,

including visiting medical students, and those individuals with whom students interact during the medical education program. A medical school develops effective written policies that address violations of the code, has effective mechanisms in place for a prompt response to any complaints, and supports educational activities aimed at preventing inappropriate behavior. Mechanisms for reporting violations of the code of professional conduct are understood by medical students, including visiting medical students, and ensure that any violations can be registered and investigated without fear of retaliation. (LCME 2017, p. 4)

In the late 1980s, Brancati (1989) traced the initial articulation of the term "pimping" to William Harvey in London in 1628. When Harvey found that his students lacked knowledge about the circulation of blood, he notably stated: "They know nothing of Natural Philosophy, these pin-heads. Drunkards, sloths, their bellies filled with Mead and Ale. O that I might see them pimped!" (p. 89). In 1889, the German microbiologist Robert Koch recorded a series of "Pumpfrage" or "pimp questions" he would use on his rounds in Heidelberg while teaching students (Brancanti 1989, p. 89). Abraham Flexner, the 20th-century reformer of medical education, observed Sir William Osler at Johns Hopkins in 1916, and later stated that he (Osler) "riddles house officers with questions like a Gatling gun" (Brancanti 1989, p. 89). Flexner also noted that William Henry Welch, the first dean of Johns Hopkins Medical School, shared that students described the questioning method as "pimping." Brancati defined pimping as "whenever an attending poses a series of very difficult questions to an intern or student. Pimp questions should come in rapid succession and should be essentially unanswerable" (Brancati 1989, p. 89).

More recently, Detsky (2009) offers a more benign view of pimping, noting that pimping can be seen as a mechanism to promote retention of knowledge. He even provides suggestions for the "pimper" (teacher) and the "pimpee" (student). For the "pimper," he suggests:

> Respect the educational order, that is, start at the bottom of the "educational chain." For example, ask the third- or fourth-year student before moving to the resident. Never ask a medical student to respond to a question after a resident has answered incorrectly. Do not embarrass other attending physicians by asking them a question unless you are sure they know the answer. However, if oth-

ers may know more about the topic than the attending physician, they can be asked for comments.

Use opportunities to encourage the uncomfortable learner to participate in the dialogue by asking them easy questions first. Stating that you do not expect anyone to answer the questions can help create a less stressed learning environment.

Use public apology in a situation where a student may have inadvertently been embarrassed.

Find an opportunity to provide praise publicly or privately; for example, a round of applause after a good presentation or giving a learner a compliment (Detsky 2009).

While some students prefer to be addressed and questioned by teachers, others may feel they are being pimped. Detsky (2009) highlights the dilemmas students face and provides advice for the "pimpees," or students, to protect against being pimped, including:

Avoidance—evade visual contact with the teacher and try to stay in the background.

The Muffin—deliberately take a bite of food; teachers will generally not ask you to speak with a full mouth.

The Hostile Response—respond to pimping questions with a tone and body language that indicates that you do not appreciate being pimped.

The List—when a list of various students' responses is being compiled, just repeating someone else's answer can be helpful.

Honorable Surrender—simply tell the teacher that you are uncomfortable being put on the spot.

Pimp Back—if circumstances allow, ask the teacher a question in return.

The Politician's Approach—when faced with an uncomfortable question, confidently answer a slightly different question.

Use of Personal Digital Assistant or Mobile Device—pull up answers in real time on a mobile device.

Do Not Sulk/Cry—remember not to get discouraged or lose composure in such situations, and remember that teachers rarely remember if a student gave a wrong answer (Detsky 2009).

Despite the long history of pimping in medical education, the majority of publications on pimping are opinion pieces, with a few evidence-based studies on the topic. A survey of fourth-year medical students' opinions on pimping revealed the hierarchical nature of pimping: both attending physicians and residents pimp students, while residents only pimp students (Wear et al. 2005). Most students placed pimping strategies into two opposing styles: "malignant" and "benign," or simply "bad" and "good" pimping (Wear et al. 2005, p. 186). Students felt comfortable, if not excited and motivated to learn more and pay closer attention to their patients, when faced with "good" pimping. Even students less enthusiastic about pimping noted its value when done by inspiring, nonthreatening teachers, and found they had become more confident when pimped (Wear et al. 2005). Another study reports the type of medical teaching preferred among students during a radiology elective (Zou et al. 2011). As part of a 90-minute radiology conference held for third- and fourth-year medical students, the educators incorporated two methods of teaching interchangeably for an equal amount of time. The first method was a didactic and traditional lecture format, while the second required student interaction and active participation in a question-and-answer session. Educators posed questions either to an entire small group, with one representative giving the collective answer, or in the larger group setting, to all students, open to anyone who volunteered to answer. During the process, professors deliberately singled out some students to answer questions, a method they defined as pimping. Following the educational experience, the students filled out survey questions. Survey results showed that 81 percent of students preferred an interactive dialogue to traditional lectures. Seventy-two percent of students noted that being pimped was an effective way to learn, but 66 percent of students preferred a volunteer-based system of answering questions. Students' definitions of pimping varied, with 46 percent of the students defining it as "attending physicians singling one person out in a group and asking question after question" (Zou et al. 2011, p. 255) and 50 percent defining it as "attending physicians singling one person out in a group to answer a question, and then moving on to someone else if he/she does not know the answer" (Zou et al. 2011, p. 255).

We can safely conclude that if pimping involves a series of esoteric, unanswerable questions fired at a learner in order to humiliate, then it is harmful; but if educators use pimping as a pedagogical method where a clinically experienced teacher poses a medical question to learners in the setting of ward rounds, in the operating room, or other small-group settings, then pimping can facilitate learning. In fact, this type of education benefits students in their growth and maturity as professionals, since they will face times when they have to answer questions in stressful circumstances (Healy and Yoo 2015). We can classify pimping as benign or malignant based on the intent and approach. If the intent is to intimidate, to establish a hierarchy, or to show off knowledge, then it is malignant pimping. If the intent is to educate and impart medical knowledge, stimulate critical thinking, or to evaluate the performance level of the learner in a sensitive way, then it is benign pimping, which learners describe as valuable.

Socratic Questioning

Socrates, the fourth-century philosopher, as documented by his student Plato, used questioning to guide students toward determining their own knowledge (Carlson 2017). Arguably, pimping is not in the spirit of Socrates' teaching method. Socrates' teaching sessions encouraged introspection and dialogue, while pimping involves one-on-one focused questioning. Socratic teaching encourages group learning, connecting new knowledge to existing knowledge, while pimping may involve a display of knowledge establishing a hierarchal order. Socratic questions are probing, leading the learner to make connections, whereas pimping questions are factual and may involve rote memorization or lists. True Socratic teaching involves asking a question with a purpose and leading learners first to a point of uncertainty where they question their own thoughts and knowledge, then to deep learning (Carlson 2017). The Socratic method encourages collaborative group dialogue, through a process that requires the student to explore their knowledge of the subject and to reinforce their position, resulting in durable understanding of the issue and the acknowledgement of the limitations of their own knowledge (Stoddard and O'Dell 2016; Healy and Yoo 2015). Socratic learning is bidirectional: both the teacher and the learner question their own thoughts and knowledge. Therefore, the approach Socrates employed with his students did not involve teaching with humiliation, and pimping would certainly not be his philosophy of teaching (Brancati 1989).

Conceptual Framework

In medical education, the teacher's role should be able to guide the learner to reach competency or proficiency in the profession. Part of the process of reaching proficiency is taking factual knowledge to a level of synthesis through application in solving problems (Mylopoulos and Regehr 2009). Questioning is a way to engage inquiry and critical thinking while promoting life-long learning and, as noted by Long et al. (2015), "questioning can engage learners by stimulating active participation in the learning process, guide them toward the understanding of deeper concepts, promote peer-peer collaboration, and build their confidence" (p. 406). We can use several frameworks to study the pedagogical impact of questioning to stimulate learning, including adaptive expertise, mind-set cognitive dissonance, and constructivism theories (Yeager and Dweck 2012; Aparicio and Rodriguez Moneo 2005; Bloom 1956; Brown et al. 1989; Goodin and Stein 2009; Festinger 1957; Skinner 2011).

Adaptive expertise theory involves how learners solve new problems through practice using their past knowledge foundation and experiences (Dyche and Epstein 2011; Mylopoulos and Regehr 2009). Guiding students in the methods of adaptive expertise early in their education helps them to develop a comfort with uncertainty and to creatively adapt to solving the problem at hand—an imperative skill in the development of a physician (Simpson et al. 1986). The mind-set theory notes that what students need the most is not self-esteem boosting, but rather a mind-set that accepts challenges they can take on and overcome (Yeager and Dweck 2012). The cognitive constructivism theory aims to guide the learner in assimilating new information using existing knowledge (Aparicio and Rodriguez Moneo 2005; Piaget 1968). The cognitive dissonance theory notes that learners have a natural tendency to seek consistency in their thoughts and behaviors (Festinger 1957). Learners experience discomfort when they encounter a conflict in their attitudes, thoughts, or behavior. Festinger (1957) refers to the discomfort or tension resulting from such a discrepancy as cognitive dissonance. Cognitive dissonance leads learners to attitudes that facilitate acquiring new information. As learners progress through medical education, they may encounter dissonance and discomfort at several points. Their response to dissonance can be irrational and limiting, or it can inspire growth in the effort to regain balance.

Health profession educators can use these theories to guide them as they endeavor to develop learners with a sense of curiosity and self-guided learning, and with the ability to adapt to new circumstances while using prior knowledge. Questioning learners can instill curiosity, which can help them later as they develop skills for innovative problem solving (Dyche and Epstein 2011; Mylopoulos and Regehr 2009). Bringing about some cognitive dissonance by using questioning at bedside or in small-group sessions (but not teaching with the intent to humiliate) can help learners develop a mind-set of resilience. It can also help learners develop knowledge through assimilation and accommodation using active discovery and dialogue (Weidman and Baker 2015).

Care of the Learner

Clinician-educators often question learners while listening to the extended narrative-history process the learners are presenting. This practice is not just an important part of the diagnostic process, but is also an integral part of educators' relationship with learners, as it helps guide the learners in knowledge development, critical thinking, and clinical judgment (Goodin and Stein 2009). Francis W. Peabody, a prominent physician, researcher, and educator at Harvard University, noted in a 1926 speech to medical students at Harvard:

> Time, sympathy and understanding must be lavishly dispensed, but the reward is to be found in that personal bond which forms the greatest satisfaction of the practice of medicine. One of the essential qualities of the clinician is interest in humanity, for the secret of the care of the patient is in caring for the patient. (Peabody 2015, p. 1868)

The same message applies to learners, where the "the secret of the care of the learner is in caring for the learner." Increasingly, attention is being brought to the growing dehumanization of medical practice and the impact on the therapeutic patient-physician relationship (Weissmann et al. 2006). The role of the educator is to foster knowledgeable learners with highly enhanced thinking skills who are compassionate and humanistic. Haidet and Stein (2006) discuss the impact of the relationship between teacher and learner on the learning process and ultimately the therapeutic relationship in patient care. The hidden curriculum in patient care also permeates the culture of the learning environment in medical education; for example, "the avoidance of uncertainty, intimidation, public shaming and humiliation, the treatment of students as objects . . . and deference to experts, regardless of their teaching abilities" (Haidet and Stein 2006, p. 17). Beach and Inui (2006) reframe the concept of relationship-centered care in enhancing a trusting and safe learning environment for teachers and learners. Relationship-centered care has four key principles of relationships, including:

The personhood of the participants is a part of the relationship.
Affect and emotions are key parts of relationships.
Relationships in health care have contextual reciprocal influences.
Maintaining "genuine" relationships in health care is morally valuable (Beach and Inui 2006).

We can transfer these concepts to the relationship between teacher and learner, where they are important in promoting the most effective and positive learning environment for critical thinking.

Questioning can be an important and positive method in the learning process (Beach and Inui 2006). How do educators know whether questioning is benign rather than malignant? The key word is *care*. It is important to ensure a learning environment where all participants feel safe and unthreatened by questions posed by educators. Some key points to ensure such an environment include:

Get to know your learners—know their names, their backgrounds, and their passions.
Allow your learners to know you as an educator and to understand that you are fallible.
Ensure that your learners know that when you ask a question, the purpose is to guide learning.
Never question learners to demonstrate your own knowledge or to humiliate.
Ensure that your learners understand that when you push them beyond their comfort zone, it is to help them move their learning to a higher level, to instill curiosity, and to help them develop resilience and deal with uncertainty.

Encourage the student when an answer is partially correct; guide and provide cues that help expand the knowledge toward the full correct answer (Dyche and Epstein 2011; Weissmann et al. 2006; Detsky 2009; Carlson 2017; Long et al. 2015; Reifler 2015).

Pearls from Our Faculty

We requested six faculty members at the University of Florida College of Medicine who were recognized by students over the years for excellence in teaching to provide us with "pearls regarding care of learner." These are available in Textbox 5.

Returning to Josh, our third-year medical student: Dr. Jones could have set up a time on day 1 of the rotation to get to know Josh and any other learners on the team. He should have discussed his educational philosophy with the students and established goals for the rotation. If Dr. Jones believes in asking students questions during rounds, he must do so in a safe environment, where learners are not fearful of giving the wrong answer.

Textbox 5. Pearls regarding the care of the learner

- Before I start working with the students, I first ask them what they want to learn. I try to incorporate that to my teaching.
- I look for teachable moments in both teaching medical knowledge and teaching resilience during my daily interaction with students.
- When I ask a question, if one student does not know, I do not go to the next student, so that the first student would feel bad. Instead, I ask a higher level learner (such as an intern).
- Care of students and care of patients is not that different.
- When I think of care of the student, I think of caring for them as a whole person, their mind-set and their personal and spiritual health.
- I want to make sure that the learners have the right resources in place—friends, family, and counselor. I am a resource too.
- In patient care situations, if the student says something wrong, I say to the patient: "Thanks for letting the student answer the questions. I want to see their views, but I wanted to teach them that I have a completely different view. Here is what I know about this topic. . . ."
- Treat the learner with respect; try not to subject the learners to what you do not want to be subjected to.

- Recognize that every learner has different learning needs. Some learners like to be challenged and put on the spot, while others do not. Some are experiential learners; others are book learners. Try to offer them a learning environment that suits their needs.
- You have to let a learner struggle a little. If you are not emotionally stimulated, then you are not learning. The challenge is to create an environment where learners are not comfortable but still safe.
- You never make anyone feel stupid. I tell the learners: If I make you feel stupid the first time I ask you the question, then I am a jerk. If you do not know the same question two days in a row, then there is a problem.
- I joke a lot so they do not feel the hierarchy. I would tell the learner: if you do not know the answer, just "phone a friend" like they do in game shows on TV.
- Sometimes, instead of just questioning them, I encourage them to think things through.
- If they seem nervous presenting a case, I joke with them. I tell the student, "I know you have a wonderful story to tell, I really want to hear it. Here are your notes; you can still look at them. But come on, tell me the story."

Compiled by authors.

Final Thoughts

As teachers, we should create an environment that nurtures curiosity, provides a comfort with uncertainty and not knowing the answer, and instills the desire to learn more through self-guided learning. Pimping is a word that elicits strong feelings and it is associated with student mistreatment and burnout. On the other hand, "good" pimping, without the negative connotations, may enable students to develop resilience and to be able to think under pressure. Ultimately, the emphasis has to be on caring for the student. Caring, however, does not mean just being gentle and sensitive; it means having the student's best interest at heart (Healy and Yoo 2015). Sometimes it is in the best interest of the learner to be in an environment that creates some degree of dissonance, allowing them to grow by learning to resolve dissonance. In the Socratic spirit, we propose renaming pimping, a colloquial term, to "transformative questioning," which has a positive connotation and encompasses the desire of educators to question students with the purpose of growth and care for the learner.

Questions for Future Research

Areas for future research include:

Does cognitive dissonance created through questioning facilitate the development of resilience?

Can faculty be trained to utilize questioning while maintaining a safe learning environment?

Do learners retain information longer when they have been questioned about a topic?

Acknowledgments

Special thanks to Drs. Carolyn Stalvey, Melanie Hagen, George Sarosi, Sanda Tan, Christina Shaw, and Daniel Rubin for their quotes and thoughts, which greatly enriched the content of this chapter.

References

Aparicio, J. J., and Rodriguez Moneo, M. (2005). Constructivism, the so-called semantic learning theories, and situated cognition versus the psychological learning theories. *Spanish Journal of Psychology* 8(02): 180–198. doi: 10.1017/s1138741600005060.

Association of American Medical Colleges (AAMC). (2016). Medical School Graduation Questionnaire 2016, All Schools Summary Report. Retrieved July 17, 2017, from https://www.aamc.org/download/464412/data/2016gqallschoolssummaryreport.pdf.

Beach, M. C., and Inui, T. (2006). Relationship-centered care. A constructive reframing. *Journal of General Internal Medicine* 21(S1): S3–8. doi: 10.1111/j.1525–1497 .2006.00302.x.

Bloom, B. S. (1956). *Taxonomy of educational objectives. The classification of educational goals: Cognitive domain.* New York: Longman.

Borkett-Jones, H., and Morris, C. (2010). Managing the trainee in difficulty. *British Journal of Hospital Medicine* 71(5): 286–289. doi: 10.12968/hmed.2010.71.5.47911.

Brancati, F. L. (1989). The art of pimping. *JAMA* 262(1): 89–90. doi: 10.1001/jama.262.1.89.

Brown, J. S., Collins, A., and Duguid, P. (1989). Situated cognition and the culture of learning. *Educational Researcher* 18(1): 32–42. doi: 10.2307/1176008.

Carlson, E. R. (2017). Medical pimping versus the Socratic method of teaching. *Journal of Oral and Maxillofacial Surgery* 75(1): 3–5. doi: 10.1016/j.joms.2016.09.019.

Detsky, A. S. (2009). The art of pimping. *JAMA* 301(13): 1379–1381. doi: 10.1001/ jama.2009.247.

Dyche, L., and Epstein, R. M. (2011). Curiosity and medical education. *Medical Education* 45(7): 663–668. doi: 10.1111/j.1365–2923.2011.03944.x.

Dyrbye, L. N., Thomas, M. R., and Shanafelt, T. D. (2006). Systematic review of depression, anxiety, and other indicators of psychological distress among U.S. and Canadian medical students. *Academic Medicine* 81(4): 354–373. doi: 10.1097/00001888-200604000-00009.

Festinger, L. (1957). *A theory of cognitive dissonance.* Evanston, IL: Row, Peterson.

Frank, E., Carrera, J. S., Stratton, T., Bickel, J., and Nora, L. M. (2006). Experiences of belittlement and harassment and their correlates among medical students in the United States: Longitudinal survey. *BMJ* 333(7570): 682. doi: 10.1136/bmj.38924.722037.7c.

Goodin, H. J., and Stein, D. (2009). The use of deliberative discussion to enhance the critical thinking abilities of nursing students. *Journal of Public Deliberation* 5(1).

Haidet, P., and Stein, H. F. (2006). The role of the student-teacher relationship in the formation of physicians. The hidden curriculum as process. *Journal of General Internal Medicine* 21(S1): S16–20. doi: 10.1111/j.1525–1497.2006.0210s1001_3.x.

Hays, R. B., Lawson, M., and Gray, C. (2011). Problems presented by medical students seeking support: A possible intervention framework. *Medical Teacher* 33(2): 161–164. doi: 10.3109/0142159x.2010.509415.

Healy, J. M., and Yoo, P. S. (2015). In defense of "pimping." *Journal of Surgical Education* 72(1): 176–177. doi: 10.1016/j.jsurg.2014.06.012.

Hinson, J. P., Griffin, A., and Raven, P. W. (2011). How to support medical students in difficulty: Tips for GP tutors. *Education for primary care: An official publication of the Association of Course Organisers, National Association of GP Tutors, World Organisation of Family Doctors* 22(1): 32–35.

Liaison Committee on Medical Education (LCME). (2017). Functions and Structure of a Medical School: Standards for Accreditation of Medical Education Programs Leading to the MD Degree. Retrieved July 5, 2017, from http://lcme.org/publications/.

Libman, M. (2002). Through the student's eyes: On pimping. *Virtual Mentor* 4(7). doi: 10.1001/virtualmentor.2002.4.7.prsp2–0207.

Long, M., Blankenburg, R., and Butani, L. (2015). Questioning as a teaching tool. *Pediatrics* 135(3): 406–408. doi: 10.1542/peds.2014–3285.

McCarthy, C. P., and McEvoy, J. W. (2015). Pimping in medical education. *JAMA* 314(22): 2347–2348. doi: 10.1001/jama.2015.13570.

Merriam-Webster OnLine (n.d.). S.v. "pimping." Retrieved July 11, 2017, from https://www.merriam-webster.com/dictionary/pimping.

Mylopoulos, M., and Regehr, G. (2009). How student models of expertise and innovation impact the development of adaptive expertise in medicine. *Medical Education* 43(2): 127–132. doi: 10.1111/j.1365–2923.2008.03254.x.

Peabody, F. W. (2015). The care of the patient. *JAMA* 313(18): 1868. doi: 10.1001/jama.2014.11744.

Piaget, J. (1968). *Six psychological studies* (A. Tenzer, trans.). New York: Knopf. (Original work published 1964).

Reifler, D. R. (2015). The pedagogy of pimping: Educational rigor or mistreatment? *JAMA* 314(22): 2355–2356. doi: 10.1001/jama.2015.14670.

Scott, K. M., Caldwell, P. H., Barnes, E. H., and Barrett, J. (2015). "Teaching by humiliation" and mistreatment of medical students in clinical rotations: A pilot study. *Medical Journal of Australia* 203(4): 185e. doi: 10.5694/mja15.00189.

Simpson, D. E., Dalgaard, K. A., and O'Brien, D. K. (1986). Student and faculty assumptions about the nature of uncertainty in medicine and medical education. *Journal of Family Practice* 23(5): 468–472.

Skinner, B. F. (2011). *About behaviorism.* New York: Vintage Books.

Stoddard, H. A., and O'Dell, D. V. (2016). Would Socrates have actually used the "Socratic method" for clinical teaching? *Journal of General Internal Medicine* 31(9): 1092–1096. doi: 10.1007/s11606-016-3722-2.

Vogan, C. L., Mckimm, J., Da Silva, A. L., and Grant, A. (2014). Twelve tips for providing effective student support in undergraduate medical education. *Medical Teacher* 36(6): 480–485. doi: 10.3109/0142159x.2014.907488.

Wear, D., Kokinova, M., Keck-Mcnulty, C., and Aultman, J. (2005). Pimping: Perspectives of 4th Year medical students. *Teaching and Learning in Medicine* 17(2): 184–191. doi: 10.1207/s15328015tlm1702_14.

Weidman, J., and Baker, K. (2015). The cognitive science of learning. *Anesthesia & Analgesia* 121(6): 1586–1599. doi: 10.1213/ane.0000000000000890.

Weissmann, P. F., Branch, W. T., Gracey, C. F., Haidet, P., and Frankel, R. M. (2006). Role modeling humanistic behavior: Learning bedside manner from the experts. *Academic Medicine* 81(7): 661–667. doi: 10.1097/01.acm.0000232423.81299.fe.

Wolf, T. M., Scurria, P. L., and Webster, M. G. (1998). A four-year study of anxiety, depression, loneliness, social support, and perceived mistreatment in medical students. *Journal of Health Psychology* 3(1): 125–136. doi: 10.1177/135910539800300110.

Yates, J., and James, D. (2006). Predicting the "strugglers": A case-control study of students at Nottingham University Medical School. *BMJ* 332(7548): 1009–1013. doi: 10.1136/bmj.38730.678310.63.

Yeager, D. S., and Dweck, C. S. (2012). Mindsets that promote resilience: When students believe that personal characteristics can be developed. *Educational Psychologist* 47(4): 302–314. doi: 10.1080/00461520.2012.722805.

Zou, L., King, A., Soman, S., Lischuk, A., Schneider, B., Walor, D., . . . Amorosa, J. K. (2011). Medical students' preferences in radiology education: A comparison between the Socratic and didactic methods utilizing PowerPoint features in radiology education. *Academic Radiology* 18(2): 253–256. doi: 10.1016/j.acra.2010.09.005.

9

Teaching Humility and Avoiding Hierarchy

JASON S. FROMM, ROBERT S. EGERMAN, AND REBECCA R. PAULY[1]

A fructibus cognoscitur arbor—The tree is known by its fruit.

Source unknown

In this chapter we discuss how the hidden curriculum can promote institutional hierarchy, which can impact interactions with learners, patients, and other health care professionals. A framework of hierarchy leading to power differentials is described and contrasted with a framework to promote humility. The chapter also provides strategies to prevent power differentials and promote humility.

Objectives

Develop an awareness of the bases of power and hierarchy in institutional, doctor-patient, teacher-learner, and interprofessional education settings.

Appraise humility as a construct for self-improvement in medicine.

During my intern year, my attending asked me to call in a consult to a subspecialty team. This particular subspecialty had a culture of being aggressive and rude. I was a bit nervous, but made the call while my attending was still with us in the team room. The fellow on call was being rude and demanded to know why I thought it essential for them to see this patient. My attending must have realized what the nature of the conversation was, as he asked to speak with the fellow. It never fails to amaze me how the

1   Jason S. Fromm, M.D., University of Florida College of Medicine, Gainesville, FL.
    Robert S. Egerman, M.D., F.A.C.O.G., University of Florida College of Medicine, Gainesville, FL.
    Rebecca R. Pauly, M.D., University of Missouri–Kansas City School of Medicine, Kansas City, MO.

tone of the conversation changes when they realize that they are talking to an attending physician. There was a complete transformation of the fellow's behavior.

I have learned the meaning of humility from one of my mentors. Over the years that I have known her, she has never mentioned the number of publications or leadership positions she has under her belt. She always responds to my requests for help, sharing all resources and information she may have. She will go out of her way to make introductions and promote my interests.

In these days of aggressive self-assertion, when the stress of competition is so keen and the desire to make the most of oneself so universal, it may seem a little old-fashioned to preach the necessity of humility, but I insist. . . .

Sir William Osler (1906, as cited in Coulehan 2010, p. 200)

The term "hidden curriculum" in medical education describes "the commonly held 'understandings,' customs, rituals, and taken-for-granted aspects of what goes on in the life-space we call medical education" (Hafferty 1998, p. 404). Educators model many values as part of the hidden curriculum, including efficiency, integrity, patient care, and teamwork (Bandini et al. 2015). Recent studies have shown that the hidden curriculum contributes to the development of professionalism and impacts the identity formation of medical students (Hendelman and Byszewski 2014; Karnieli-Miller et al. 2011). Unfortunately, the hidden curriculum in medical education often promotes egoism and a sense of personal entitlement. The years of grueling training, along with their economic impact, lead to a sense of entitlement, lack of humility, and arrogance—although justified pride in accomplishments should not diminish humility (Coulehan 2010). Additionally, a heavy clinical workload and lack of support are often factors contributing to rude and dismissive behavior among trainees and practicing physicians (Bradley et al. 2015). In the United States, the Institute of Medicine (2001) published the report "Crossing the Quality Chasm: A New Health System for the 21st Century," which recommends that "health professionals should be educated to deliver patient centered care as members of an interdisciplinary team" (p. 79).

This chapter discusses the impact of hierarchy and power differential as part of the hidden curriculum and describes humility as a construct in health care.

Hierarchy and Power Differentials

The issues related to hierarchy and power are rarely discussed in medical education. Health care professionals have the opportunity to exert power in their day-to-day activities. Patient care, with all the complexities of health care delivery, is saturated with interactions between providers of different power levels. This includes teacher-learner, doctor-patient, and interprofessional interactions. In the absence of reflection, these interactions can result in cynicism, curtness, and even burnout.

Conceptual Framework of Power

Social psychologist Raven (2008) proposes a conceptual framework to understand power. The primary bases of power he describes include:

Legitimate or positional power: Power or influence exerted because of a person's position, for example, a doctor in an administrative or supervisory role, such as a hospital executive or department chair.

Expert and informational power: Power based on knowledge and expertise, for example, a subspecialist attending physician.

Reward and coercive power: The influence exerted by a person in power who can decide rewards and penalties or can threaten negative consequences, for example, a faculty supervisor or department chair.

Referent power: Power based on a person's charisma, or the force of personality. Often, a leader displaying referent power not only creates policy but also embodies it, for example, a dean or provost known for their charisma.

Awareness of and reflection on these bases of power help health professionals model behaviors that can lead to a transformative leadership style, which incorporates and expands power strategies into a principles-driven, relationship-oriented leadership approach (Gabel 2012). Hierarchy and power differentials impact not just individuals but also groups or sets of people. The social dominance theory examines the social and psychological process contributing to the formation and maintenance of social hierarchies (Pratto et al. 1994). It brings to light how one group can exert power over another group through economic advantage, nationality, race, religion, or gender. In medicine, social dominance comprises the implicit control of norms and institutional or individual culture by the more powerful individual or group—the teacher in a learner/instructor setting, or administrative heads at the faculty and institutional level (Pratto et al. 1994). As an example, in academic medicine, social dominance by men faculty leads to barriers in the advancement of women in academic medicine (Conrad et al. 2010). While both men and women faculty view hierarchy negatively, women faculty describe the hierarchy as a factor impacting their career advancement (Conrad et al. 2010). Additionally, hierarchizing specialties based on the level of prestige can impact medical students' career choices (Lepièce et al. 2016).

Institutional culture of hierarchy

Institutional hierarchy results in mistreatment of individuals throughout their careers. In 2012, in the American Association of Medical Colleges Graduation Questionnaire, 47 percent of medical students had been mistreated in one or more situations (Mavis et al. 2014). Another survey reports an 83 percent prevalence of mistreatment of medical students; 64 percent were mistreated by a faculty member and 75 percent by a trainee/resident (Cook et al. 2014). Mistreatment correlates with poor emotional and mental health and leads to burnout (Haviland et al. 2011; Lubitz and Nguyen 1996). In a survey of doctors in the United Kingdom, 31 percent described being subject to rude, dismissive, and aggressive behavior, and 40 percent stated that this behavior moderately to severely affected their working day (Bradley et al. 2015). Still other studies have noted that disruptive, demeaning, disrespectful behavior is often directed to those at the bottom of the totem pole (Leape et al. 2012). There is ample evidence that people in positions of power can and do abuse their power. Notably, however, we must not equate rude and dismissive behavior with bullying, which is a pattern of abuse that persists over time (Bradley et al. 2015).

Teacher-learner hierarchy

Models describing the impact of hierarchy highlight the importance of three factors: perceived power distance, leader inclusiveness, and psychological safety (Appelbaum et al. 2016). Power distance is the way individuals perceive the unequal distribution of status and power within organizations. Leader inclusiveness encompasses leaders' openness and availability as well as their acknowledgement of contributions by individuals. An environment with reduced power distance and increased leadership inclusiveness positively impacts psychological safety. Psychological safety is the comfort with which lower ranking members of a team can voice opinions without exposing themselves to negative consequences. A low level of safety may contribute to a low rate of adverse event reporting (Appelbaum et al. 2016).

Medical hierarchy is prevalent, and has the potential to undermine and contradict humility. However, a transformative team leader can cultivate an environment where questioning is welcome (Appelbaum et al. 2016). Lowering learners' risk from disclosing errors is likely to increase reporting (Appelbaum et al. 2016). In addition, cultivating an institutional culture of valuing humility as a personal and professional trait can be an effective strategy to counter hierarchy and power issues (Gruppen 2015).

Doctor-patient hierarchy

Power dynamics play a role in the doctor-patient relationship as well. Shared decision making is essential for effective health care; however, patients must have the knowledge required to guide decisions and the power to participate (Joseph-Williams et al. 2014). Patients need to be encouraged to think about and express personal values while making medical decisions, and practitioners need to examine their own preconceptions about patient involvement. Philosopher Michel Foucault is known for his theories on the relationship of power and knowledge and how it is used as a form of social control in society (Foucault 1984). He developed the theory of the "medical gaze," describing the separation of the patient (as a person) from the disease. According to his theory, the practice of medicine was dehumanized when physicians viewed the human body only as a source of information for pathophysiology and disease. He noted the importance of addressing power issues in the physician-patient relationship and advocated for the physician's gaze to treat both mind and body problems. Even today the patient often assumes a submissive state while the physicians discuss the treatment (Forbat et al. 2009). Patients may also enter unspoken contracts with physicians, characterized by passive behavior, compliance, and endorsing the prevailing view that "doctor knows best" (Joseph-Williams et al. 2014, p. 17). We must foster a culture in which physicians empower patients to abandon such silent contracts and join in shared decision-making conversations.

Interprofessional hierarchy

Health care professionals are usually educated in separate institutions, colleges, or disciplines. This system results "interdisciplinary dissonance: the separate training and administration of professionals who are expected to work as a unit" (Lingard et al. 2002, p. 733). The model helps ensure that basic competencies are achieved for each of the professions, but it results in health professionals training in silos, with the expectation that they will work in teams later. In the United States, the Institute of Medicine (2001) recommends that health profession education be designed to provide patient-centered care in interdisciplinary teams. Some institutions have introduced interprofessional education (IPE) for collaborative learning within the health care work force (Blue et al. 2010). Hawkes et al. (2013) note a positive change in attitudes toward different health professionals after working together in IPE interventions for at least seven weeks. Graduates from programs offering IPE note that there is often little social contact between different professions, even when they are located at the same university (Gilligan et al. 2014). While on rotations, students interacted only while seeing patients together and maintained social silos. Students spoke only of functional aspects of working together and described their experience as "bland" (p. 7). In Europe, educational institutions have established clinical interprofessional education wards, where undergraduate students from the medicine, nursing, physiotherapy, and occupational therapy programs participate in interprofessional patient care in teams (Hallin et al. 2009). Researchers note that such interventions improve understanding of other professions and positively impact communication skills (Hallin et al. 2009), but are less able to positively influence attitudes and perceptions toward other professions (Hammick et al. 2007).

Health care has traditionally placed a gender divide between medicine and nursing; decision making and management skills are associated with physicians, and nurturing care with nurses (May and Fleming 1997). Despite the advancement of women in health care, these stereotypes persist (Langendyk et al. 2015). Health profession education also instills strong occupational identities, which contribute to maintaining such stereotypes and hierarchy within disciplines (Langendyk et al. 2015).

As Gilligan et al. (2014) note, "When-ever undergraduates who are taught best practice skills in communication, teamwork and interprofessional practice graduate and work in a climate of hierarchy, silos and stereotypes, any IPE efforts are destined to fail" (p. 8).

Humility

Roots of humility in medicine

The Hippocratic Oath emerged after Hippocrates' death in the 5th century B.C., and has been modified by medical schools over centuries. It continues to represent ideal physician behavior. At the University of Florida College of Medicine, the modified Hippocratic Oath mentions humility twice (Textbox 6): first to remind us to honor the people whose illnesses have provided a source for medical learning and discovery, and second to prompt us to be humble in our daily medical practices. In order to ensure that such Hippocratic Oaths serve as living documents, institutions need to remind practitioners of their oath, revisit the contents of the oath, and provide strategies to learn humility. Gruppen (2015) calls for humility to be treated as a value that needs to be learned and practiced. We must continually remind learners and practitioners about the importance of humility in interpersonal interactions as well as intellectual humility, that is, respect for different points of views (Gruppen 2015).

Dr. Jacobs has had a busy on-call night at the hospital. Upon entering a patient's room, she has difficulty completing her examination, as there is a shrill beeping sound coming from the next bed in the shared room. The source of the noise is a bed alarm. The patient in the next bed would like a cool cloth to place on his forehead to relieve a headache and nausea. As the nurse had not responded, the patient was attempting to get up, which triggered the bed alarm. Dr. Jacobs enquires what the patient needs, then takes a fresh washcloth from the closet, runs it under cold water, wrings it out, and places it on the forehead of her patient's roommate. After she finishes seeing her patient, she finds the adjacent patient's nurse and informs her that the patient was not feeling well.

In his writings on humility and respect in medical education, Gruppen (2015) suggests that drawing attention to humility in academic culture can assist in the adoption of quality improvement initiatives. In the above vignette, Dr. Jacobs had recently completed training at an institution with a patient care initiative called "No passing while the light is flashing." The catchy phrase, paired with a memorable graphic placed throughout the hospital wards, was a reminder that all workers are responsible for addressing patient safety and needs. Dr. Jacobs could have chosen to ignore the alert or passed it on to another care provider, but she went one step further, displaying humility while meeting a patient's needs.

Textbox 6. University of Florida College of Medicine modified Hippocratic Oath

In the presence of family, friends, teachers, and colleagues, and in the spirit of Hippocrates, I pledge to keep this oath.

First, I will do no harm.

I will honor those who taught me the art and science of medicine.

I will remember with gratitude and humility those whose illness or injury provided examples from which I learned, and, in their honor, I will continue the pursuit of knowledge.

I will share my knowledge with future colleagues and all who are in want or need of it.

I will practice medicine with conscience and humility, and I will act with enduring respect for the dignity of human life. Foremost in my mind will be compassion, respect, and impartial care for my patients.

I will hold sacred the trust of my patients and respect the secrets that they confide in me.

I will not be swayed by greed, prejudice, or selfish ego in the practice of my art.

Finally, I will do all in my power to help my patients reach physical, mental, and spiritual health, and I will strive for this balance in my own life.

May I have the courage and character to hold these principles sacred from this day forward as I place myself into the service of humankind. This oath I make solemnly, freely, and upon my honor.

Printed with permission of the Medical Education Office, College of Medicine, Gainesville, Florida.

Conceptual Framework for Humility

Coulehan (2010) provides a conceptual framework for humility, describing humility in medicine as a virtue consisting of:

Constant self-awareness: Having confidence in what one knows while accepting limitations, particularly while caring for patients with complicated medical or social problems

Empathic openness to others: the ability to understand or feel others' pain

An appreciation of, and the gratitude for, the privilege of caring for others (Coulehan 2010).

Humility may have negative connotations of being "wishy-washy" or "weak" (Coulehan 2010). Society and the media contribute to this perception as they depict doctors as being always in charge, confident, and often arrogant. In reality, humility is an attribute of strength and self-awareness in a complex health care environment rather than a characteristic of meekness or indecisiveness. Others argue that humility should serve as a "crowning virtue" as it indicates courageous willingness to recognize one's own limitations (DuBois et al. 2013). In contrast, arrogance or lack of humility prevents physicians from recognizing failure and impacts their ability to respond to feedback. Coulehan (2010) describes four personal attributes that constitute humility:

Unpretentious openness, or the capacity for introspection and assessing personal strengths and weaknesses.

Avoidance of arrogance by reflecting and avoiding self-entitlement behavior and "rough, blustering" manners.

Honest self-disclosure, which seems straightforward—the duty to acknowledge an error, for example, is not controversial in today's world—but in practice, physicians may either compartmentalize the truth or restrict the amount of detail they openly acknowledge.

Modulation of self-interest, or balancing altruism as a doctor with a reflective awareness of personal limitations; similar conceptually to the "Golden Mean" theory of Aristotle's times: the desirable middle between two extremes.

Describing her journey through academic medicine as an individual with a rare disease, spondyloepiphyseal dysplasia, neonatologist Dr. Jennifer Arnold notes that "the ability to have humility as a physician is not only a sign of a good doctor, but it can be one of the most challenging attributes to maintain" (Arnold 2013, p. 332). She suggests posing the following question to one's self and, if the response to any of the questions is yes, reflecting on the courage to be humble:

> Do you take opportunities to claim credit for things that you are involved in, regardless of the level of your involvement?
> Do you like to be right and to prove what you know?
> Do you think your role as a physician is more important than the role of another, such as a janitor, teacher, or politician?
> Do you believe you are capable of handling things on your own, without help from others?
> Do you ever brag about things you do or can do? (Arnold 2013).

Humility and leadership

Morris et al. (2005) associate humility in leaders with authentic, servant, and transformative leadership styles. Authentic leaders have a high degree of self-awareness and acknowledge their limitations. Service leaders "operate out of a motivational basis of 'I serve' as opposed to 'I lead'" (Morris et al. 2005, p. 1339). Transformational leaders have a vision for the future, engaging and inspiring others to work together. Notably, as a construct for leadership, humility may be less effective in individualist vs. collectivist cultures, in high vs. low power distance cultures, and in masculine vs. feminine cultures (Morris et al. 2005).

Humility and Cultural Competence Curriculum

The U.S. population is growing increasingly diverse. According to the U.S. Census Bureau, nonwhites will make up 56 percent of population in 2060: Hispanics/Latinos, 28 percent; African Americans, 14 percent; Asians Americans, 9 percent; American Indian and Alaska Native, 1.3 percent; and mixed races, 6 percent (Colby and Ortman, 2015; U.S. Census Bureau 2016). Health professionals must achieve cultural competence to be able to treat an increasingly heterogeneous patient population. Previously, static issues like ethnicity, race, gender, age, income, education, sexual orientation, ability, and faith defined culture. New definitions of culture include sets of competing discourses and practices, within situations characterized by the unequal distribution of power (Kumagai and Lypson 2009). Researchers have suggested that cultural humility should be integrated into cultural competency training (Chang et al. 2012). Based on the work of Chinese philosophers, the QIAN curriculum emphasizes the role of humility as part of cultural competence in order to build the doctor-patient relationship. The curriculum highlights the importance of:

Questioning—self-questioning and critique
Immersion—bidirectional immersion in another's culture
Active listening
Negotiation flexibility—negotiation of mutually acceptable alternates (Chang et al. 2012).

Final Thoughts

Several institutions have employed strategies to prevent or counter mistreatment (Mavis et al. 2014). Role-playing exercises increase sensitivity and awareness of mistreatment. Other reflective activities focus on awareness and offer the learner an opportunity to express their experiences in a safe and constructive environment. Journaling, team-based ethics cases, cultural competency training, and mindfulness of implicit biases all work to combat low self-esteem (Jennings 2009). Other strategies include mandatory training programs and rewards recognizing exemplar residents and faculty (Fried et al. 2012). The Yale School of Medicine holds an annual "Power Day," when medical students and nursing students define and analyze power dynamics (Angoff et al. 2016). The university invites guest speakers, offers small group exercises, and recognizes residents that use power positively with Power Day Awards. Researchers note that the intervention promotes dialogue about power, fosters interprofessional relationships, and helps reward positive role modeling (Angoff et al. 2016).

The World Health Organization and the Institute of Medicine have identified interprofessional education (IPE) as a strategy to promote an interdependent working relationship (Buring et al. 2009). IPE can play an important role in countering hierarchy in the workplace (Smith et al. 2015). The term "professional equipoise" describes the suspension of one's own assumptions regarding members of other allied health professions, which can help professionals appreciate the value of the contributions of other professions (Smith et al. 2015). Smith et al. describe four essential elements for the deliberate practice of IPE: committing together to the superordinate goal of providing high-functioning interprofessional care; suspending judgment, or taking on a "beginners mind" (professional equipoise); treating one another with respect; and encouraging inquisitiveness about one another's training and profession (Smith et al. 2015, p. 607).

It is important for all health care professionals to appreciate and understand how they conceptualize power and make behavioral changes. Cultivating humility is a challenging, but necessary, mechanism to prevent both mistreatment and hierarchy. Humility can help negate the effects of power. Methods to develop humility include:

Recognizing the limitations of one's own knowledge and experience

Placing oneself in the shoes of the learner, colleague, or patient

Maintaining an open viewpoint and learning others' perspectives

Addressing others in a friendly, noncondescending tone

Reminding oneself that it is a privilege to be able to help others.

Medical educators should consider incorporating statements to assess humility in the definition of professionalism, including unpretentious openness, honest self-disclosure, avoidance of arrogance, and modulation of self-interest (Coulehan 2011).

In the first vignette at the start of the chapter, we see an interaction between an intern and a fellow (trainee in a subspecialty). There is an obvious power differential: typically, the fellows have a few more years of training under their belts, and may exploit their "positional power." Junior doctors are more likely to be exposed to rude and dismissive behavior, whereas senior doctors are treated with more respect due to their status, seniority, and position in the hierarchy (Bradley et al. 2015). Interventions described above, such as "power days," mandatory training sessions, and building institutional cultures of respect and humility, can prevent such negative interactions and improve resiliency. The second vignette provides an example of the impact of a leader displaying humility. Such leadership cultivates an environment that promotes positive interactions and helps decrease burnout.

In this chapter, two contrasting frameworks are presented—a framework to help readers recognize power differentials (Raven 2008) and a framework to promote humility (Coulehan 2010). Power differentials in several settings—institutional, doctor-patient, teacher-learner, and IPE—are discussed. Strategies to consciously cultivate humility can be a powerful tool for health care educators in each of the settings.

Questions for Future Research

Further studies are needed to:

Develop and evaluate programs that create awareness of humility and power.

Describe programs to counter mistreatment and the impact those programs have on future behavior. In evaluating the impact on behavior, researchers should include questions assessing how trainees and faculty handle power dynamics, and should provide feedback to close the loop.

Publish examples of role plays and vignettes for others to use while developing awareness sessions.

Examine the impact of culture on the relationship of humility and leadership.

Explore the impact of interventions to learn and practice humility.

References

Angoff, N. R., Duncan, L., Roxas, N., and Hansen, H. (2016, 03). Power day: Addressing the use and abuse of power in medical training. *Journal of Bioethical Inquiry* 13(2): 203–213. doi: 10.1007/s11673-016-9714-4.

Appelbaum, N. P., Dow, A., Mazmanian, P. E., Jundt, D. K., and Appelbaum, E. N. (2016). The effects of power, leadership and psychological safety on resident event reporting. Medical Education 50(3): 343–350. doi: 10.1111/medu.12947.

Arnold, J. L. (2013, 05). Humility in medicine. *Clinics in Dermatology* 31(3): 332–335. doi: 10.1016/j.clindermatol.2012.11.003.

Bandini, J., Mitchell, C., Epstein-Peterson, Z. D., Amobi, A., Cahill, J., Peteet, J., . . . Balboni, M. J. (2015, 11). Student and faculty reflections of the hidden curriculum: How does the hidden curriculum shape students' medical training and professionalization? *American Journal of Hospice and Palliative Medicine* 34(1): 57–63. doi: 10.1177/1049909115616359.

Blue, A. V., Mitcham, M., Smith, T., Raymond, J., and Greenberg, R. (2010, 08). Changing the future of health hrofessions: Embedding interprofessional education within an academic health center. *Academic Medicine* 85(8): 1290–1295. doi: 10.1097/acm.0b013e3181e53e07.

Bradley, V., Liddle, S., Shaw, R., Savage, E., Rabbitts, R., Trim, C., . . . Whitelaw, B. C. (2015, 11). Sticks and stones: Investigating rude, dismissive and aggressive communication between doctors. *Clinical Medicine* 15(6): 541–545. doi: 10.7861/clinmedicine.15-6-541.

Buring, S. M., Bhushan, A., Broeseker, A., Conway, S., Duncan-Hewitt, W., Hansen, L., and Westberg, S. (2009, 09). Interprofessional education: Definitions, student competencies, and guidelines for implementation. *American Journal of Pharmaceutical Education* 73(4): 59. doi: 10.5688/aj730459.

Chang, E., Simon, M., and Dong, X. (2012, 05). Integrating cultural humility into health care professional education and training. *Advances in Health Sciences Education* 17(2): 269–278. doi: 10.1007/s10459-010-9264-1.

Colby, S. L., and Ortman, J. M. (2015). *Projections of the size and composition of the U.S. population: 2014 to 2060.* Current Population Reports, P25-1143. Washington, D.C.: U.S. Census Bureau.

Conrad, P., Carr, P., Knight, S., Renfrew, M. R., Dunn, M. B., and Pololi, L. (2010, 04). Hierarchy as a barrier to advancement for women in academic medicine. *Journal of Women's Health* 19(4): 799–805. doi: 10.1089/jwh.2009.1591.

Cook, A. F., Arora, V. M., Rasinski, K. A., Curlin, F. A., and Yoon, J. D. (2014, 05). The prevalence of medical student mistreatment and its association with burnout. *Academic Medicine* 89(5): 749–754. doi: 10.1097/acm.0000000000000204.

Coulehan, J. (2010, 08). On humility. *Annals of Internal Medicine* 153(3): 200–201. doi: 10.7326/0003-4819-153-3-201008030-00011.

Coulehan, J. (2011). "A gentle and humane temper": Humility in medicine. *Perspectives in Biology and Medicine* 54(2): 206–216. doi: 10.1353/pbm.2011.0017.

Dubois, J. M., Kraus, E. M., Mikulec, A. A., Cruz-Flores, S., and Bakanas, E. (2013, 07). A humble task: Restoring virtue in an age of conflicted interests. *Academic Medicine* 88(7): 924–928. doi: 10.1097/acm.0b013e318294fd5b.

Forbat, L., Maguire, R., McCann, L., Illingworth, N., and Kearney, N. (2009, 02). The use of technology in cancer care: Applying Foucault's ideas to explore the changing dynamics of power in health care. *Journal of Advanced Nursing* 65(2): 306–315. doi: 10.1111/j.1365-2648.2008.04870.x.

Foucault, M. (1984). *The Foucault reader: An introduction to Foucault's thought.* P. Rabinow (ed.). London: Penguin Books.

Fried, J. M., Vermillion, M., Parker, N. H., and Uijtdehaage, S. (2012, 09). Eradicating medical student mistreatment: A longitudinal study of one institution's efforts. *Academic Medicine* 87(9): 1191–1198. doi: 10.1097/acm.0b013e3182625408.

Gabel, S. (2012, 11). Power, leadership and transformation: The doctor's potential for influence. *Medical Education* 46(12): 1152–1160. doi: 10.1111/medu.12036.

Gilligan, C., Outram, S., and Levett-Jones, T. (2014, 03). Recommendations from recent graduates in medicine, nursing and pharmacy on improving interprofessional education in university programs: A qualitative study. *BMC Medical Education* 14(1). doi: 10.1186/1472-6920-14-52.

Gruppen, L. D. (2015, 01). Competency-based education, feedback, and humility. *Gastroenterology* 148(1): 4–7. doi: 10.1053/j.gastro.2014.11.021.

Hafferty, F. W. (1998, 04). Beyond curriculum reform: Confronting medicine's hidden curriculum. *Academic Medicine* 73(4): 403–407. doi: 10.1097/00001888-199804000-00013.

Hallin, K., Kiessling, A., Waldner, A., and Henriksson, P. (2009, 01). Active interprofessional education in a patient based setting increases perceived collaborative and professional competence. *Medical Teacher* 31(2): 151–157. doi: 10.1080/01421590802216258.

Hammick, M., Freeth, D., Koppel, I., Reeves, S., and Barr, H. (2007, 01). A best evidence systematic review of interprofessional education: BEME Guide no. 9. *Medical Teacher* 29(8): 735–751. doi: 10.1080/01421590701682576.

Haviland, M. G., Yamagata, H., Werner, L. S., Zhang, K., Dial, T. H., and Sonne, J. L. (2011, 07). Student mistreatment in medical school and planning a career in academic medicine. *Teaching and Learning in Medicine* 23(3): 231–237. doi: 10.1080/10401334.2011.586914.

Hawkes, G., Nunney, I., and Lindqvist, S. (2013, 04). Caring for attitudes as a means of caring for patients—improving medical, pharmacy and nursing students' attitudes to each other's professions by engaging them in interprofessional learning. *Medical Teacher* 35(7): e1302–1308. doi: 10.3109/0142159x.2013.770129.

Hendelman, W., and Byszewski, A. (2014, 07). Formation of medical student professional identity: Categorizing lapses of professionalism, and the learning environment. *BMC Medical Education* 14(1). doi: 10.1186/1472-6920-14-139.

Institute of Medicine. (2001). *Crossing the quality chasm: A new health system for the 21st century*. (2001). Washington, D.C.: National Academy Press.

Jennings, M. L. (2009, 10). Medical student burnout: Interdisciplinary exploration and analysis. *Journal of Medical Humanities* 30(4): 253–269. doi: 10.1007/s10912-009-9093-5.

Joseph-Williams, N., Elwyn, G., and Edwards, A. (2014, 03). Knowledge is not power for patients: A systematic review and thematic synthesis of patient-reported barriers and facilitators to shared decision making. *Patient Education and Counseling* 94(3): 291–309. doi: 10.1016/j.pec.2013.10.031.

Karnieli-Miller, O., Vu, T. R., Frankel, R. M., Holtman, M. C., Clyman, S. G., Hui, S. L., and Inui, T. S. (2011, 03). Which experiences in the hidden curriculum teach students about professionalism? *Academic Medicine* 86(3): 369–377. doi: 10.1097/acm.0b013e3182087d15.

Kumagai, A. K., and Lypson, M. L. (2009, 06). Beyond cultural competence: Critical consciousness, social justice, and multicultural education. *Academic Medicine* 84(6): 782–787. doi: 10.1097/acm.0b013e3181a42398.

Langendyk, V., Hegazi, I., Cowin, L., Johnson, M., and Wilson, I. (2015, 06). Imagining alternative professional identities: Reconfiguring professional boundaries between nursing students and medical students. *Academic Medicine* 90(6): 732–737. doi: 10.1097/acm.0000000000000714.

Leape, L. L., Shore, M. F., Dienstag, J. L., Mayer, R. J., Edgman-Levitan, S., Meyer, G. S., and Healy, G. B. (2012, 07). Perspective: A culture of respect, part 1: The nature and causes of disrespectful behavior by physicians. *Academic Medicine* 87(7): 845–852. doi: 10.1097/acm.0b013e3182583536.

Lepièce, B., Reynaert, C., van Meerbeeck, P., and Dory, V. (2015, 05). Social dominance theory and medical specialty choice. *Advances in Health Sciences Education* 21(1): 79–92. doi: 10.1007/s10459-015-9612-2.

Lingard, L., Reznick, R., Devito, I., and Espin, S. (2002, 08). Forming professional identities on the health care team: Discursive constructions of the "other" in the operating room. *Medical Education* 36(8): 728–734. doi: 10.1046/j.1365-2923.2002.01271.x.

Lubitz, R. M., and Nguyen, D. D. (1996, 02). Medical student abuse during third-year clerkships. *JAMA* 275(5): 414–416. doi: 10.1001/jama.275.5.414.

Mavis, B., Sousa, A., Lipscomb, W., and Rappley, M. D. (2014, 05). Learning about medical student mistreatment from responses to the medical school graduation questionnaire. *Academic Medicine* 89(5): 705–711. doi: 10.1097/acm.0000000000000199.

May, C., and Fleming, C. (1997, 05). The professional imagination: Narrative and the symbolic boundaries between medicine and nursing. *Journal of Advanced Nursing* 25(5): 1094–1100. doi: 10.1046/j.1365-2648.1997.19970251094.x.

Morris, J. A., Brotheridge, C. M., and Urbanski, J. C. (2005, 10). Bringing humility to leadership: Antecedents and consequences of leader humility. *Human Relations* 58(10): 1323–1350. doi: 10.1177/0018726705059929.

Pratto, F., Sidanius, J., Stallworth, L. M., and Malle, B. F. (1994). Social dominance orientation: A personality variable predicting social and political attitudes. *Journal of Personality and Social Psychology* 67(4): 741–763. doi: 10.1037//0022-3514.67.4.741.

Raven, B. H. (2008, 09). The bases of power and the power/interaction model of interpersonal influence. *Analyses of Social Issues and Public Policy* 8(1): 1–22. doi: 10.1111/j.1530-2415.2008.00159.x.

Smith, C. S., Gerrish, W. G., Nash, M., Fisher, A., Brotman, A., Smith, D., . . . Dreffin, M. (2015, 11). Professional equipoise: Getting beyond dominant discourses in an interprofessional team. *Journal of Interprofessional Care* 29(6): 603–609. doi: 10.3109/13561820.2015.1051216.

United States Census Bureau (U.S. Census Bureau). (2016). QuickFacts: United States. Retrieved from https://www.census.gov/quickfacts/table/PST045216/00.

SECTION III

Implications for Teaching

10

A Framework for Discussing Controversial Topics in Medical Education

RYAN NALL, LAUREN SOLBERG,
ROBERT L. COOK, AND BRENDA ROGERS[1]

Ductus exemplo—Lead by example.
Source unknown

We use Lawrence-Wilkes and Ashmore's model of rational reflective enquiry as a framework for navigating controversial topics, such as guns and abortions, in the clinical setting with learners. Through the use of controversial topics where opposing beliefs are held, we provide a guide for educational discussions to inform and enhance the understanding of different perspectives.

Objectives

Provide a framework for discussing controversial topics in the clinical setting with learners.

Improve communication on controversial topics with learners.

John is a third-year medical student who sees Austin, a 5-year-old boy brought in to the clinic by his mother and father for a well-child exam. John finds Austin is in good health and meeting his developmental milestones. John counsels the family about home safety but decides not to

---

1   Ryan Nall, M.D., University of Florida College of Medicine, Gainesville, FL.
    Lauren Solberg, J.D., M.T.S., University of Florida College of Medicine, Gainesville, FL.
    Robert L. Cook, M.D., M.P.H., University of Florida College of Medicine, Gainesville, FL.
    Brenda Rogers, M.D., F.A.A.P., F.A.C.P., University of Missouri–Kansas City School of Medicine, Kansas City, MO.

ask about guns in the home, as he believes this is not any of his business. He recalls some states have enacted legislation prohibiting doctors from inquiring about guns in the home, and is uncertain regarding the laws in his state. John exits the exam room and presents the case to you. You are the attending physician, and you routinely ask families about gun safety. When you ask John if he discussed guns in the home with the family, he states he did not.

Nicole, a third-year medical student, is working with you, the attending physician, in clinic. She sees Anna, a 29-year-old single woman with no children, who came into clinic alone. Anna tells Nicole she took a home pregnancy test five days ago that was positive. She tells Nicole now is not a good time for her to have a baby. Anna recalls the date of her last menstrual period was at least eight weeks ago, but she does not know an exact date. Anna does not have an OB/GYN since she regularly sees you to perform her annual exams. She tells Nicole she wants to talk today about terminating the pregnancy. Nicole is opposed to pregnancy termination in all cases, except where the health or life of the mother is at risk. You do not perform abortions, however; you refer patients to abortion providers when your patients request this service.

We live in an increasingly interconnected world that developed, through multinational trade agreements, international businesses, and Internet connectivity, into a global village (Schwarz 2001). Physicians and learners from different countries and ethnic traditions now train and care for patients together (Schwarz 2001). Teachers, learners, and patients bringing diverse values to the learning environment challenge the traditional model of teacher-learners as expert-novice (Kumagai and Lypson 2009). In *The World Is Flat*, Friedman (2005) describes how the world now functions as a global collaborative practice to provide excellence in knowledge, efficiency, and quality to each other. This also applies to the practice of caring for patients, and teaching learners. As we confront our ability to work together globally, we confront the challenges this new opportunity provides. Even within the United States, learners come from different socioeconomic, ethnic, geographical, and/or religious traditions, which frame how they will care for patients. This creates a challenge when learners, educators, and patients have differing values related to their health care.

Kumagai and Lypson (2009) argue that we must go beyond cultural competency to foster a critical consciousness "of the self, others, and the world and a commitment to addressing issues of societal relevance in health care" in learners (p. 782). Many of these "issues of societal relevance" are controversial and heavily value-laden. Yet medical educators cannot ignore these issues with their learners, and learners should feel comfortable exploring them in an academic environment. Educators who recognize the importance of critical consciousness use societal, cultural, and historical information as a frame of reference in encouraging learners to consider holistically a multitude of problem-solving options (Kumagai and Lypson 2009). Identifying and encouraging the use of critical consciousness in problem solving require a different approach to education. They require collaboratively and nonjudgmentally discussing specific topics and situations with the goal of understanding multiple perspectives about the topic, and focusing on an effective discussion as opposed to focusing on a specific outcome as a measure of competency. Frambach and Martimianakis (2016) note:

> awareness of a patient's personal history and community; of social determinants of health; of power structures and how they impact health and health-care systems; and, most importantly, social action and transformation resulting from this awareness . . . cannot simply be translated into neatly, described, measurable competencies. (p. 1)

The hierarchical nature of the physician-learner relationship in the educational setting tends to lead both parties to avoid controversial and uncomfortable topics such as politics, spiritual beliefs, or personal values. Despite your best intentions to be respectful, at some point, a need will arise to address a controversial topic where there is a difference of opinion. However, if educators do not recognize that a topic is controversial, they will fail to reinforce important points about it. Others may be so afraid of the controversy surrounding a topic they avoid it entirely. Hess (2005) describes these and other approaches teachers take when faced with a controversial topic.

Denial: Teacher denies that a topic is controversial.
Privilege: Teacher teaches toward a particular perspective.

Avoidance: Teacher avoids discussion of the topic.

Balance: Teacher includes different perspectives in discussion.

Although using the balance approach is optimal, Hess (2005) notes there are problems in its application. When a difference of opinion arises, educators must acknowledge the difference's existence, and strive to understand the other's opinion, before they can more effectively argue for their viewpoint (Hess 2005).

Halman et al. (2017) review the use of critical consciousness in health professional education and summarize common practices of a critical pedagogy that include promoting authentic dialogue, inviting stories, questioning the status quo, and challenging the power hierarchy. In using critical consciousness to educate learners, educators encourage them to consider why a particular approach to problem solving exists, and then question whether an alternative approach might be more effective. Creating a supportive and encouraging environment where all participants freely share their own opinions allows everyone to contribute their respective personal experiences and values to the conversation. Both Kumagai and Lypson (2009) and Hess (2005) describe this environment as the goal of exercising critical consciousness.

We introduce Lawrence-Wilkes and Ashmore's (2014) model of rational reflective enquiry as the framework for achieving Kumagai and Lypson's (2009) and Hess's (2005) goals in navigating controversial topics, such as guns and abortions, that arise in the clinical setting. We chose these controversial health-related topics due to the opposing beliefs held by different individuals and societal organizations. Nationally, each topic has been the center of debate, demonstrating the polarity of beliefs and the passion of those who voice their opinions. Fundamentally, the objective of this chapter is to improve communication with learners to allow them to become better informed and more capable of discussing controversial topics with others (including patients) who may not share their viewpoint.

Background: Guns in the United States

In the United States, gun rights and regulations have been a source of fervent debate throughout the country's history:

1791: The Second Amendment of the U.S. Constitution protects the right to bear arms stating, "A well-regulated militia, being necessary to the security of a free state, the right of the people to keep and bear arms, shall not be infringed" (U.S. Const., Amend. II).

1934: Seeking to regulate firearms in response to the era's gangster culture, Congress passed the National Firearms Act of 1934 ("History of gun-control legislation" 2012). This act placed a tax on the production of machine guns, banned the ownership of sawed-off shotguns, and required recording firearms sales in a national registry (National Firearms Act of 1934).

1968: On the heels of the assassination of John F. Kennedy, Robert Kennedy, and the Rev. Martin Luther King, Jr., the U.S. Congress passed the Omnibus Crime Control and Safe Streets Act of 1968 and the Gun Control Act of 1968 ("History of gun-control legislation" 2012). The bills prohibited the sale of firearms to all convicted felons, drug users, and the mentally ill, and raised the minimum age to purchase handguns from a federally licensed dealer to 21 ("History of gun-control legislation" 2012).

1986: In response to concerns that the federal government was abusing its power in enforcing gun laws, Congress passed the Firearm Owners Protection Act of 1986 ("History of gun-control legislation" 2012). This law protected gun dealers from repeated inspection and banned a federal registry of gun ownership ("History of gun-control legislation" 2012).

1993: Congress passed the Brady Handgun Violence Prevention Act, which mandates background checks of gun buyers in order to prevent sales to people prohibited from owning guns under the 1968 legislation ("History of gun-control legislation" 2012).

2005: Congress passed the Protection of Lawful Commerce in Arms Act, which granted gun manufacturers immunity from civil lawsuits filed over crimes committed with firearms ("History of gun-control legislation" 2012).

Despite ongoing debate, no further major federal legislation has been passed.

In 2014, 33,599 Americans died of gunshot wounds, and on October 1, 2017, the United States suffered the worst mass shooting in its history

(National Center for Health Statistics 2017). In response, the American Medical Association called the frequent mass shootings in the United States a public health crisis and advocated for lifting the CDC ban on gun violence research ("AMA Calls Gun Violence 'A Public Health Crisis'" 2016). Since 2010, the number of guns manufactured in the United States nearly doubled, to 10.9 million in 2013 (Horsley 2016). Surprisingly, despite the increase in manufacturing, the number of households with guns has fallen from 50 percent in the 1970s to 31 percent in 2015 (Horsley 2016). Nonetheless, firearm-related deaths continue to be one of the top three causes of death among American youth (Heron 2016). The number of accidental deaths in children due to firearms is difficult to ascertain because of mislabeling as suicides or homicides (Luo and McIntire 2013). Between 1979 and 1997, one study identified 30,000 unintentional firearm deaths, of which 4,600 were children under the age of 15 (Miller et al. 2001). The authors also found that states with stronger safe gun storage policies had lower rates of unintentional gun deaths (Miller et al. 2005). Furthermore, brief office-based counseling by pediatricians has increased the safe storage of firearms by parents (Barkin et al. 2008).

Background: Abortion in the United States

In 1973, the Supreme Court of the United States held in *Roe v. Wade* that state laws criminalizing abortion unnecessary to save the life of the mother regardless of the stage of pregnancy violate the due process clause of the Fourteenth Amendment of the U.S. Constitution (*Roe v. Wade* 1973). Although the U.S. Constitution does not explicitly identify a right to privacy, the Supreme Court read this right into the Fourteenth Amendment in *Roe v. Wade* and extended it to women who seek to terminate their pregnancies (*Roe v. Wade* 1973). Consequently, abortion is legal in all 50 states and the District of Columbia. In 1992, in *Planned Parenthood v. Casey*, the Supreme Court introduced a new framework for abortion rights, opining that prior to viability, a state may regulate abortions, but not impose an "undue burden" on women who seek to terminate the pregnancy (*Planned Parenthood v. Casey* 1992). After viability, however, a state may regulate and indeed prohibit abortion except where necessary for the health or life of the mother (*Planned Parenthood v. Casey* 1992). This case also established that any law that has the purpose or effect of "plac[ing] a substantial obstacle in the path of a woman seeking an abortion before the fetus attains viability" presents an undue burden and is unconstitutional (*Planned Parenthood v. Casey* 1992).

What constitutes an "undue burden" continues to be a hotly debated topic, and further ligation is likely. In 2016 in *Whole Woman's Health v. Hellerstedt*, the Supreme Court held that Texas state law requiring abortion providers to have admitting privileges at hospitals near their abortion clinics and requiring abortion clinics to meet ambulatory surgical center standards imposes an undue burden (*Whole Woman's Health v. Hellerstedt* 2016). Future cases may consider whether, for example, certain waiting periods or mandatory ultrasounds also meet the standard (Wis. Stat. § 253.10(3g) 2017); Woman's Right to Know Act of 2002, 2017).

Despite its legalization, abortion remains a controversial topic because religious, educational, and personal experiences influence an individual's views (Pew Research Center 2009). Advocates for increased access to abortion underscore a woman's right to make her own reproductive decisions and cite the increased likelihood of women undergoing unsafe procedures—and the resulting health risks—when abortion is illegal or restricted (Committee on Health Care for Underserved Women 2014b). To support their views, opponents of abortion and advocates of additional restrictions on abortion cite the fetus's rights; psychological risks to the woman, such as regret, depression, and suicide; and the protection of the health of the woman (Jesudason and Weitz 2015).

The abortion controversy arises in several ways in the clinical setting. Upon learning she is pregnant, a patient may ask a physician about her options, request a referral for pregnancy termination, or ask a physician to terminate her pregnancy. Ultimately, even when not directly confronted with one of these scenarios, a physician is likely to encounter patients in their care who have had an abortion; the Guttmacher Institute reports 30 percent of women in the United States will have had an abortion by the age of 45 (Guttmacher Institute 2017).

Conceptual Framework

Lawrence-Wilkes and Ashmore (2014) propose a model for reflective rationalism (Figure 7) that provides the foundation for discussing controversial topics in medical education.

Reflection is central in navigating these topics for both teacher and learner. Lawrence-Wilkes and Ashmore argue that this reflective process

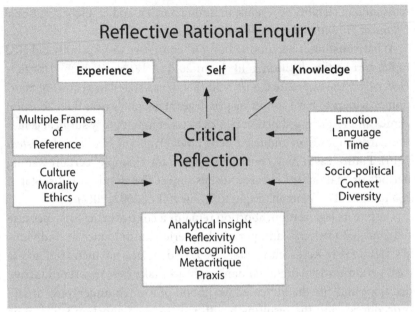

Figure 7. Reflective rational enquiry. Printed with permission. From L. Lawrence-Wilkes and L. Ashmore, *The reflective practitioner in professional education*. New York: Palgrave Macmillan, 2014.

informs by "reflecting in through intrapersonal self-reflection and reflecting out through interpersonal social interactions" (2014, p. 63). Intrapersonal self-reflection accounts for different worldviews, culture, morality, ethics, emotion, language, sociopolitical context, and diversity. This in turn informs the practitioner's sense of self, experience, and knowledge through social interaction. Furthermore, this framework recommends engaging in metacognition—considering how we think about challenging topics, and metacritique—actively analyzing how we appraise our actions. Thus, critical reflection plays a key role in interpreting our interactions, developing our own position, and eventually acting—a process Lawrence-Wilkes and Ashmore (2014) refer to as praxis.

While Lawrence-Wilkes and Ashmore's model does not specifically address teaching controversial topics (2014), we posit its application to improve communication between learners and medical educators surrounding controversial topics. We emphasize the role of intrapersonal and interpersonal reflection (Figure 7) through the application of their framework. We feel that better communication informs learners and increases their capacity to engage in conversations about controversial topics with patients or colleagues who have differing perspectives.

Applying the Framework

1. Recognize the teachable moment

A teachable moment presents itself each time you see a patient with a learner, but arguably more so when there is an emotionally charged issue. This is true regardless of whether you share the same views as your learner or your patient. Many educators choose to avoid these topics; however, evasion teaches the learners the unintended lesson that they should avoid these conversations with colleagues and patients.

Vignette 1 represents a teachable moment for reflection where the educator shares his or her knowledge with the learner on the often-divisive issue of guns. Despite the widespread impact of gun violence, physicians rarely screen or counsel patients about guns (Wintemute et al. 2016; Butkus and Weissman 2014). Many barriers exist to physician screening and counseling, including education on what to say during screening (Butkus and Weissman 2014). A survey of pediatric residency program directors reported that only one-third of programs offered training on firearm counseling (Price 1997). Physicians also report concerns about damaging the patient relationship (Walters et al. 2012), and that screening infringes on patients' rights (Price et al. 2013). Educators can use teachable moments to inform learners about ways to handle firearm counseling in a given situation despite differences in their beliefs.

Vignette 2 presents the controversial topic of abortion which, despite its prevalence, often has minimal presence in medical education curricula. However, learners value education about abortion in both preclinical and clinical curricula (Espey et al. 2005; Espey et al. 2008); moreover, the American College of Obstetrics and Gynecology advocates for its inclusion in medical school curricula (Committee on Health Care for Underserved Women 2014a). Given the paucity of abortion education in medical schools and the likelihood that a woman will seek an abortion or have had an abortion during her lifetime, discussion about abortion is a teachable moment.

2. Stop and listen to the learner

Medical educators can be quick to offer guidance and advice to learners blindly. In controversial topics, it is important to first stop and listen to the learner's understanding and beliefs of the case. In many nonclinical learning environments, content is controlled, but this is not always the case in the clinical setting—which is both the beauty and the challenge of clinical medical education. Often we do not know what we will encounter when we enter the patient's room. The Yale Center for Teaching and Learning recommends establishing clear ground rules for discussing controversial topics (Yale Center for Teaching and Learning 2016). When we stop and listen, we set not only the tone, but also the ground rules for the discussion. We show the learner respect and allow for curiosity in their opinion. With a deeper understanding of the learner's beliefs and knowledge on the subject, we move the conversation forward in an informed manner. When we stop and listen, we also need to check our own emotions on the subject, as well as acknowledge the learner's.

In no way should a learner's personal feelings on a controversial topic affect his or her performance evaluation or grade. Settings of higher education, including the clinical setting, are safe environments where respectful discussion and questioning occurs. Explicitly state to learners that you welcome the chance to discuss their personal views, that their opinions do not affect their grades, and that your goal is to help them recognize and understand the issue from multiple perspectives. Thus, you will discuss multiple viewpoints in order to be comprehensive in your discussion.

In vignette 1, stopping and listening to John's perspective on screening for firearms—whether based on personal belief, classroom knowledge, or other information—is critical. Ask John why he did not ask questions about firearm ownership, and listen to his response. When we understand John's perspective, we can then tailor teaching points, address any confusion, and possibly become more informed if the student has more knowledge or experience. Consider the following:

> *Does John feel we should not be performing firearm screening?* If John is concerned about invasion of privacy regarding firearm possession, you can discuss how to broach sensitive topics with patients. Then, John can apply this strategy to other topics beside firearms. *What is John's knowledge base on the subject?* If John is very knowl-

edgeable about firearms or gun safety, or owns a firearm, then sharing his knowledge is beneficial to you and the family. Conversely, if John has misinformation or no information about firearm use, storage, or safety, then you can take this opportunity to share relevant medical society guidelines.

How has John's prior experience affected his current viewpoint? John's personal experience regarding firearms—either positive or negative—affects his viewpoint. Discussion about his experience provides another learning opportunity.

Discussing these questions and others that might arise becomes an opportunity to research, review, and discuss personal recommendations and national policies.

In vignette 2, you and Nicole have contrasting views of abortion. This is common. Areas of agreement or disagreement may include whether it is ethical to perform abortions, whether it is appropriate to counsel patients about an option for terminating a pregnancy, and whether a physician opposed to abortion is compelled to refer a patient to another physician for counseling or for the procedure itself.

You can understand what drives Nicole's beliefs by stopping and listening to her. Although Nicole may be reluctant to share her personal beliefs about this controversial topic, she may in fact be comfortable having an open discussion. You can inform her that you want to discuss several perspectives on the issue of abortion to allow for a robust conversation in which you each attempt to understand alternative views. If you stop and listen, Nicole may provide you with some cues about what she wants or needs to learn about this topic. A young woman residing in the United States is most likely exposed to discussions surrounding abortion. Listening to how Nicole developed her opinions provides an opportunity to discuss resources and review relevant literature. In addition, our patients obtain information from resources that are unfamiliar to us. By listening to Nicole, we can learn how students and our patients gather information for decision making. You provide Nicole with a method to approach controversial topics when discussing how to locate and identify resources, and to use them in developing opinions. This demonstrates to her an objective approach in assessing information that is not aimed at changing her opinion. Moreover, it is difficult to detect how sensitive a topic like abortion is to Nicole if you do not stop and listen.

3. Take a step back (use controversy constructively)

Once you understand the learner's knowledge base and beliefs, it is important to take a step back and examine the context and facts of the case. Describing arguments on both side of a controversial issue helps broaden the learner's knowledge on the issue (Burkstrand-Reid et al. 2011). Further, context is critical. If you did not observe the interaction between the patient and the learner, taking time to understand the factors that went into their responses adds to your understanding.

Now you have an opportunity to take an alternative stance. If the learner is willing, ask them to defend a different viewpoint in a continued discussion; then, after you have shared opinions and information, switch positions. This exercise compels both of you to understand and respect alternative stances, recognizing there might be a small piece of credibility to an opinion with which you disagree. It requires a broad review of the literature in search of information supporting the opposite position. This defense of an opposing position benefits the doctor-patient relationship. Implementing structured debates where residents argued a viewpoint that was not necessarily congruent with their own position improved rates of discussion with patients regarding mammography screening before age 50 (Helenius et al. 2006).

In vignette 1, reviewing the current state law governing screening and counseling for firearms as well as national professional guidelines on the topic is paramount to John's education. For example, Massachusetts does not have a law prohibiting screening and counseling, and the American Academy of Pediatrics endorses screening for firearms and counseling on firearm safety by providers (Dowd et al. 2012). By taking a step back, you can determine if John understands these state laws and professional guidelines before making a personal decision to avoid screening and counseling.

In vignette 2, since Nicole has freely shared with you her beliefs about abortion, taking a step back helps you understand where she is coming from. If her—or another learner's—beliefs, either in favor or in opposition to abortion, stem from her value system, taking a step back guides your teaching approach. The role of a medical educator is not to try to change your learners' views, but to understand them in order to reflect on how learners communicate with patients and colleagues whose values conflict with their own—and possibly with yours. However, you cannot reach this next step without listening and taking a step back to reflect on how best to approach the learner.

4. Explain your approach

After the learner understands the facts and arguments surrounding a controversial issue, and how the context of the case affects the outcome of the conversation, then you can explain your approach to the issue. You are not trying to change the learner's mind about the controversial topic; rather, you are teaching them how to care for the patient in a thoughtful way. If you or the learner feel you cannot provide the care the patient asks for, your role shifts to teaching the learner how to react in a clinical setting when a patient requests treatment that you believe you cannot provide (Orr 2013). Describing your approach to difficult clinical scenarios provides a real-life example the learner can reference in the future. However, your approach reveals your position on an issue, which could be polarizing. Therefore, it is critical to emphasize that this is your individual approach, and others might handle the scenario differently. This is the art of medicine and clinical teaching. In the book *Crucial Conversations*, the authors argue that you must "learn to look" for signs that the learner is becoming silent or shifting to a confrontational stance (Patterson et al. 2012). Such a shift in tone can destroy the learning environment. If you begin to detect this shift, pause and assess your own tone and goals for the conversation.

In the practice of medicine, we confront awkward and uncomfortable conversations or situations. Thus, you are using the topic at hand to instruct the learner on ways to participate in difficult conversations. Encouraging the learner to practice their questions during role play is helpful. The goal of the "Explain your approach" step is to allow the learner to participate in the process and find ways to meet the patient's expectations in a less uncomfortable manner. This process develops respect of personal opinions while meeting the needs of the patient.

Once you have completed your conversation and explained your approach, take the learner back into the exam room so you can address the topic with the patient and/or family. Allow the learner to observe your conversation, communication style, and actions. This demonstration gives you the opportunity to request feedback about your approach. Furthermore, it provides guidance about how the student might engage in a future conversation about a controversial topic.

In vignette 1, when you reach this step, share with John why and how you screen for firearms in the home. Provide him with the context, and compare your approach to published guidelines. Again, if your approach differs from John's, remember to respect his beliefs and "learn to look" for signs that the learning environment is being compromised (Patterson et al. 2012). If John disagrees with you, then work with him to determine alternative ways to ensure home safety regarding firearms. For example, create a written questionnaire that includes reasons for asking about firearms in the home, or develop an explanatory statement the learner verbalizes prior to asking questions. This becomes a fantastic opportunity to respect the learners' approach while modeling respectful communication on a controversial topic.

In vignette 2, share with Nicole why you refer your patients to an abortion provider after you discuss all options and that is their preference. Role-model your approach, including explanations of the governing laws in your state about abortion and why you feel Anna is a candidate for the procedure. In addition, discussing with Nicole about the prevalence of abortion and women's reasons for abortion can help Nicole contextualize Anna's request. In 2013, the Center for Disease Control indicated approximately two-thirds of abortions performed that year were within the first eight weeks of gestation; over 91 percent were within the first 13 weeks (Jatlaoui et al. 2016). Anna does not necessarily know how far along she is in her pregnancy, but her history of a positive pregnancy test five days ago suggests she is within the first 13 weeks of her pregnancy. Recent research notes that the most common reasons women cite for seeking abortions are poor timing of the pregnancy in their lives and the substantial cost of raising a child (Biggs et al. 2013). Anna's reason for pregnancy termination is similar to that of other women. Knowledge of this information lets Nicole know Anna is comparable to other patients she may encounter. In addition, it invites the discussion of how a physician communicates with a patient seeking an abortion after 13 weeks' gestation, and/or one who has a less common rationale for her request.

You are now asking Nicole to observe and understand your approach to a controversial topic. This provides an opportunity to discuss the expectations of the physician-patient relationship, and the inherent needs and expectations of that relationship. At times, those needs and expectations conflict, and adjustments occur. Ultimately, physicians have the responsibility to do what is best for the patient. A physician morally opposed to abortion who feels they cannot meet Anna's medical needs must explicitly state this to her and refer her to a physician who can. It is not morally permissible to decline care for a patient without assisting her in identifying another professional who can care for the patient. In your discussion with Nicole, including this information clarifies your approach to difficult situations beyond abortion while lessening the emotions aroused by going from a specific to a general topic. It also provides Nicole with suggestions on how a physician can assist Anna without compromising their own personal beliefs.

5. Debrief

Given the fast-paced nature of clinical medicine, the conversations outlined in this framework may not occur in their entirety at one time or in this exact order; they often demand more time than is available in a busy clinical setting. When a controversial topic arises, the medical educator recognizes its importance by letting the learner know that they will circle back to the topic later. For example, you can state, "This is an important topic and I want to make sure we have more time to discuss it. After clinic, let us sit down and discuss this topic in more depth. For now, observe my approach to this issue. Other physicians may take a different approach, but this is my approach." Providing additional time to address the issues shows the learner the topics' importance and complexity, and the learner, respect. Asking for the learner's feedback is a great starting point for the conversation. The educator can respond directly to the learner's observations and interpretations of the clinical encounter.

In vignette 1, John may feel uncomfortable about sharing his feelings about firearms in real time. Ask John to first observe your approach and conversation with the patient's parents. Circling back to the topic gives him another opportunity, after processing the discussion, to recognize this as a tough topic that arouses a wide range of personal feelings. Then ask John for his impression of your discussion with Austin's parents on firearms safety. He might express different ideas on how he would handle the discussion, which leads to a method of inquiry that is more comfortable and acceptable to him. It is important to include your reasons for your comments to the patient/family so that John completely understands your intentions, which may not seem obvious to a learner. For example, you explain that you asked whether the gun in the home was stored loaded or empty because you were seeking to provide guidance on methods of safe gun storage. The American Academy of Pediatrics (2012) recommends storing firearms unloaded and locked, and storing ammunition separately in a locked box. This illustrates that you were not being intrusive, but rather were gathering information to assist you in how best to provide safety guidance.

In vignette 2, Nicole may have additional questions for Anna, or she may need to talk about the experience. Your role is to help her feel comfortable asking those questions. Given the often emotionally charged nature of abortion, it is important to find a quiet safe place where you can discuss the case. Any reluctance Nicole may have shown to share her views may fade in such a setting. Providing a safe space for further reflection allows and encourages Nicole to think critically about the conversation, even if she remains reluctant to share her personal views or discuss the case further. When debriefing, discuss your reasons for or against offering Anna other options, for instance, adoption. The debriefing time is also a good time to discuss a relevant professional organization's approach to this controversial topic, such as the American College of Obstetrics and Gynecology's committee opinion on a physician's conscientious refusal to perform the procedure (American College of Obstetricians and Gynecologists 2007).

6. Role-model

No matter how your belief on a controversial topic compares to a learner's, you have an opportunity to role-model respectful communication and understanding of another's viewpoint throughout the entire interaction (Yale Center for Teaching and Learning 2016). This is the most important part of the learning process. As physicians, we regularly enter conversations with patients in which our views differ. Learning a respectful communication style is fundamental to a physician's development. Maintaining a nonjudgmental and respectful demeanor provides learners with an approach in discussing emotional and controversial topics effectively. The physicians in both vignettes have a wonderful opportunity to model the appropriate behavior. Refer to the chapter "Introspection about Role

Modeling" for a complete and in-depth review of the impact and process of role modeling in medical education.

Final Thoughts

Medical education continues to become more global with increasing interactions between trainees, educators, and patients from different backgrounds or unique social or cultural perspectives. This diversity is relevant not only to our clinical care, but to our perspectives on ethical or health policy issues, many of which are controversial.

We have used two case examples of controversial topics with differing perspectives of the patients, learners, and educators, and a framework, based on existing medical theories and approaches, to guide educational discussions that inform and enhance the understanding of different perspectives. It also fosters a critical consciousness in the learner. By helping learners gain more comfort in discussing controversial topics encountered in clinical care, we hope that medical educators and learners become more confident advocating for health care issues over time.

Medical schools must address the needs of a broader cultural society, and in doing so they often seek to enhance the "cultural competency" of learners. However, understanding a different culture does not lead learners to seek to improve social justice. Rather, one-on-one discussions about controversial topics provide an opportunity for instructors to facilitate exchanges rather than lecture.

Ultimately, we recognize the imperfect nature of Hess' "balanced" approach to teaching controversial topics. As she points out, learners do not view the issue as controversial (even though the teacher does), and efforts to appear balanced may in fact appear biased (Hess 2005). Furthermore, while privileging may bleed into indoctrinating (Hess 2005), the reality is that privileging in medical education is often unavoidable in a clinical setting. Unlike the classroom setting, where the teacher presents information to her learners, in the clinical setting the teacher presents information to patient and learner, and ultimately has a decision to make about the care of the patient. Denial of the controversial nature of issues like gun ownership or abortion that arise in a clinical setting disregards the political, religious, and cultural discourse surrounding them. Avoidance is common, as evidenced by the omission of abortion education from medical school curricula. Avoiding a controversial issue removes the possibility of a maximally rich learning experience. The framework we presented, in the context of guns and abortion, helps medical educators take a balanced approach to controversial topics in medicine.

Discussions of other controversial topics, such as prescribing opioid pain medications, prejudice, health care access, or contraceptives can benefit from this or a similar framework. Medical educators should not avoid these issues because of controversy. They provide educational value to the learner by serving as a platform for students to learn how to address and resolve conflict, discuss uncomfortable topics with a patient, and understand another's viewpoint (Philpott et al. 2011).

Lawrence-Wilkes and Ashmore's (2014) framework for reflective rational enquiry is a model for the critical reflection that is vital to discussing controversial topics in medical education. Navigating these conversations in clinical practice involves recognizing the teachable moment, stopping and listening to the learner, taking a step back, explaining your approach, debriefing, and role modeling throughout your interaction. This approach better informs learners and makes them more capable of discussing controversial topics with others.

Questions for Future Research

How can medical educators incorporate discussions of controversial topics into patient simulations, standardized patients, or small group discussions?

Which frameworks are most effective for discussion of controversial topics in medical education?

How are patients affected by these discussions?

References

AMA calls gun violence "a public health crisis." (2016, June 14). Retrieved from https://www.ama-assn.org/ama-calls-gun-violence-public-health-crisis.

American College of Obstetricians and Gynecologists. (2007). ACOG Committee opinion no. 385: The limits of conscientious refusal in reproductive medicine. *Obstetrics and Gynecology* 110(5): 1203–1208. doi: 10.1097/01.aog.0000291561.48203.27.

American Pediatrics Association. (2012). American Academy of Pediatrics gun violence policy recommendations. Retrieved from https://www.aap.org/en-us/advocacy-and-policy/federal-advocacy/documents/aapgunviolencepreventionpolicyrecommendations_jan2013.pdf.

Barkin, S. L., Finch, S. A., Ip, E. H., Scheindlin, B., Craig, J. A., Steffes, J., . . . Wasserman, R. C. (2008). Is office-based counseling about media use, timeouts, and firearm storage effective? Results from a cluster-randomized, controlled trial. *Pediatrics* 122(1). doi: 10.1542/peds.2007-2611.

Biggs, M. A., Gould, H., and Foster, D. G. (2013). Understanding why women seek abortions in the U.S. *BMC Women's Health* 13(1). doi: 10.1186/1472-6874-13-29.

Burkstrand-Reid, B., Carbone, J., and Hendricks, J. S. (2011). Teaching controversial topics. *Family Court Review* 49(4): 678–684. doi: 10.1111/j.1744-1617.2011.01404.x.

Butkus, R., and Weissman, A. (2014). Internists' attitudes toward prevention of firearm injury. *Annals of Internal Medicine* 160(12): 821–827. doi: 10.7326/m13-1960.

Committee on Health Care for Underserved Women. (2014a). ACOG Committee opinion no. 612: Abortion training and education. *Obstetrics and gynecology* 124(5): 1055–1059. doi: 10.1097/01.AOG.0000456327.96480.18.

Committee on Health Care for Underserved Women. (2014b). ACOG Committee opinion no. 613: Increasing access to abortion. *Obstetrics and Gynecology* 124(5): 1060–1065. doi: 10.1097/01.AOG.0000456326.88857.31.

Dowd, M.D., Sege, R. D., Council on Injury, Violence, and Poison Prevention Executive Committee, and American Academy of Pediatrics. (2012). Firearm-related injuries affecting the pediatric population. *Pediatrics* 130(5): e1416–1423. doi: 10.1542/peds.2012-2481.

Espey, E., Ogburn, T., Chavez, A., Qualls, C., and Leyba, M. (2005). Abortion education in medical schools: A national survey. *American Journal of Obstetrics and Gynecology* 192(2): 640–643. doi: 10.1016/j.ajog.2004.09.013.

Espey, E., Ogburn, T., Leeman, L., and Nguyen, T. Gill, G. (2008). Abortion education in the medical curriculum: A survey of student attitudes. *Contraception* 77(3): 205–208. doi: 10.1016/j.contraception.2007.11.011.

Frambach, J. M., and Martimianakis, M. A. (2017). The discomfort of an educator's critical conscience: The case of problem-based learning and other global industries in medical education. *Perspectives on Medical Education* 6(1): 1–4. doi: 10.1007/s40037-016-0325-x.

Friedman, T. L. (2005). *The world is flat: A brief history of the twenty-first century*. Bridgewater, NJ: Paw Prints/Baker and Taylor.

Guttmacher Institute. (2017). United States: Abortion. Retrieved from https://www.guttmacher.org/united-states/abortion.

Halman, M., Baker, L., and Ng, S. (2017). Using critical consciousness to inform health professions education. *Perspectives on Medical Education* 6(1): 12–20. doi: 10.1007/s40037-016-0324-y.

Helenius, I. M., Goldstein, C. E., Halm, E. A., and Korenstein, D. (2006, 10). Using structured debate to teach a controversial topic: Mammography for women in their 40s. *Teaching and Learning in Medicine* 18(4): 292–296. doi: 10.1207/s15328015tlm1804_3.

Heron, M. (2016) Deaths: Leading causes for 2014. *National Vital Statistics Reports* 65(5). Hyattsville, MD: National Center for Health Statistics.

Hess, D. E. (2005). How do teachers' political views influence teaching about controversial issues? *Social Education* 69(1): 47–48.

History of gun-control legislation. (2012, December 22). Retrieved from https://www.wash-ingtonpost.com/national/history-of-gun-control-legislation/2012/12/22/80c8d624-4ad3-11e2-9a42-d1ce6d0ed278_story.html?utm_term=.5e2a75594311.

Horsley, S. (2016, January 05). Guns in America, by the numbers. Retrieved from http://www.npr.org/2016/01/05/462017461/guns-in-america-by-the-numbers.

Jatlaoui, T. C., Ewing, A., Mandel, M. G., Simmons, K. B., Suchdev, D. B., Jamieson, D. J., Pazol, K. (2016). Abortion surveillance—United States, 2013. *MMWR Surveillance Summary* 65(SS-12):1–44. doi: http://dx.doi.org/10.15585/mmwr.ss6512a1.

Jesudason, S., and Weitz, T. (2015). Eggs and abortion: "Women-protective" language used by opponents in legislative debates over reproductive health. *Journal of Law, Medicine & Ethics* 43(2): 259–269. doi: 10.1111/jlme.12241.

Kumagai, A. K. and Lypson, M. L. (2009). Beyond cultural competence: Critical consciousness, social justice, and multicultural education. *Academic Medicine* 84(6): 782–787. doi: 10.1097/acm.0b013e3181a42398.

Lawrence-Wilkes, L., and Ashmore, L. (2014). *The reflective practitioner in professional education.* New York: Palgrave Macmillan.

Luo, M., and McIntire, M. (2013, September 28). Children and guns: The hidden toll. Retrieved from http://www.nytimes.com/2013/09/29/us/children-and-guns-the-hidden-toll.html?pagewanted=all&_r=0.

Miller, M., Azrael, D., and Hemenway, D. (2001). Firearm availability and unintentional firearm deaths. *Accident Analysis and Prevention* 33(4): 477–484. doi: 10.1016/s0001-4575(00)00061-0.

Miller, M., Azrael, D., Hemenway, D., and Vriniotis, M. (2005). Firearm storage practices and rates of unintentional firearm deaths in the United States. *Accident Analysis and Prevention* 37(4): 661–667. doi: 10.1016/j.aap.2005.02.003.

National Center for Health Statistics. (2017, May 03). Retrieved from https://www.cdc.gov/nchs/fastats/injury.htm.

National Firearms Act of 1934, Pub. L. 73-474474, 48 Stat. 1236, codified as amended at 26 U.S.C. §§ 5801–5872 (1934).

Orr, R. D. (2013) Autonomy, conscience, and professional obligation. *Virtual Mentor* 15(3): 244–248. doi: 10.1001/virtualmentor.2013.15.3.msoc1-1303.

Patterson, K., Grenny J., McMillan, R, and Switzler A. (2012). *Crucial conversations: Tools for talking when stakes are high.* New York: McGraw-Hill.

Pew Research Center. (2009, Oct. 1). Abortion and morality. Retrieved from http://www.pewforum.org/2009/10/01/support-for-abortion-slips5/.

Philpott S., Clabough J., McConkey L., and Turner T. (2011). Controversial issues: To teach or not to teach? That is the question! *Georgia Social Studies Journal* 1(1): 32–44.

Planned Parenthood v. Casey. 505 U.S. 833 (1992).

Price, J. H. (1997). Training in firearm safety counseling in pediatric residency programs. *Archives of Pediatrics and Adolescent Medicine* 151(3): 306–310. doi: 10.1001/archpedi.1997.02170400092016.

Price, J. H., Thompson, A., Khubchandani, J., Wiblishauser, M., Dowling, J., and Teeple, K. (2013). Perceived roles of emergency department physicians regarding anticipatory guidance on firearm safety. *Journal of Emergency Medicine* 44(5): 1007–1016. doi: 10.1016/j.jemermed.2012.11.010.

Roe v. Wade. 410 U.S. 113 (1973).

Schwarz, R. (2001). Globalization and medical education. *Medical Teacher* 23(6): 533–534. doi: 10.1080/01421590120090943.

U.S. Constitution (U.S. Const.), Amendment II.

Walters, H., Kulkarni, M., Forman, J., Roeder, K., Travis, J., and Valenstein, M. (2012). Feasibility and acceptability of interventions to delay gun access in VA mental health settings. *General Hospital Psychiatry* 34(6): 692–698. doi: 10.1016/j.genhosppsych.2012.07.012.

Whole Woman's Health v. Hellerstedt, 579 U.S. 2292 (2016).

Wis. Stat. § 253.10(3g) (2017).

Wintemute, G. J., Betz, M. E., Ranney, M. L. (2016). Yes, you can: Physicians, patients, and firearms. *Annals of Internal Medicine* 165(3): 205–213. doi: 10.7326/M15-2905.

Woman's Right to Know Act of 2002, Ala. Code § 26–23A-4 (2017).

Yale Center for Teaching and Learning. (2016). Teaching controversial topics. Retrieved from ctl.yale.edu/teaching/ideas-teaching/teaching-controversial-topics.

11

Teaching in the Electronic Era

Medical Records and Social Media

EDLIRA MASKA, ERIC I. ROSENBERG, AND DANIËLLE VERSTEGEN[1]

Tempora mutantur et nos mutamur in illis—
Times change and we change with them.

Ovid

In this chapter we discuss the benefits and challenges that educational institutions face in using electronic health records (EHR). We discuss challenges related to social media, including ethical and legal challenges in a medical education, providing educational approaches for consideration in the EHR and social media era.

Objectives

Introduce current applications of electronic health records (EHR) and social media in health care and medical education.

Recognize the benefits and pitfalls of the EHR and social media.

Identify contemporary issues related to the use of EHR and social media.

A third-year medical student at a teaching hospital is assigned the task of interviewing and examining a patient in the Emergency Department (ED) who will be hospitalized. The student spends 20 minutes in a workroom

1 Edlira Maska, M.D., University of Florida College of Medicine, Gainesville, FL.

Eric I. Rosenberg, M.D., M.S.P.H., F.A.C.P., University of Florida College of Medicine, Gainesville, FL.

Daniëlle Verstegen, F.H.M.L., Department of Educational Research and Development, Maastricht University, The Netherlands.

reading about the patient's presenting complaint, history of present illness, and test results as recorded by an ED scribe. He then walks to the ED to see the patient.

A medical trainee (resident) posts an interesting case on his Facebook page with a picture of the patient that he helped take care of during rounds in a large teaching hospital. He describes in detail the patient's clinical history and his cotrainees and attendings involved in the case. The resident's Facebook page is public; thus, anyone can read the contents of his postings.

An oncology physician who has a personal blog frequently posts patients' stories. Most of these stories are heartfelt narratives of the difficult clinical and emotional course of her patients' illnesses. On her blog, she posts a description of one of her patients: "Mr S is lovely 88-years old gentleman who I have taken care of for five years. On his visits to my office, he has always accompanied by wife and often by his grandkids. Unfortunately his cancer is now Stage IV and today I admitted him to the local hospital where I have admitting privileges, for worsening shortness of breath. ... They have opted for comfort care."

Electronic Health Records and Medical Education

We live in an era where technological advancement has allowed social media and EHR to infiltrate many aspects of health care; however, little is known about the potential benefits and unintended consequences of these technologies on learners in medical education (Tierney et al. 2013). EHR systems are intended to unify the previously fragmented paper medical record and improve quality of care, while simultaneously increasing time for patient interaction and academic activities (Tierney et al. 2013). EHR systems also make it possible to share patient information among health care institutions and physicians, which could potentially improve the quality of medical care. However, researchers must evaluate concerns for patient privacy.

Medical learners start adapting to EHR early in their education to develop proficiency with the process of entering and reviewing the myriad clinical, social, and demographic data available within these systems. A cross-sectional survey of the Association of Clerkship Directors in Internal Medicine at U.S. and Canadian academic health centers showed that EHR use has become prevalent; however, many of the programs in the study did not have specific policies to address how or even if learners should be permitted to use these systems (Mintz et al. 2009). Studies cited concerns regarding compliance and productivity losses as possible justifications to restrict student access to EHR information entry (Mintz et al. 2009). Tierney et al. (2013) studied the effect of EHR on achievement of educational milestones set by the Accreditation Council for Graduate and Medical Education (ACGME). The authors emphasized the challenges that educational institutions face when implementing EHR and measuring the impact of EHR in medical education. As Tierney et al. (2013) point out, on the one hand, EHR has the potential to enhance education and develop clinical decision-making skills. It offers opportunities to teach best practices and allows for communication between in-network providers. On the other hand, the more advanced the EHR becomes, the more information can be found that is not clinically relevant or beneficial from an educational standpoint. EHRs are not standardized and their designs are highly complex, which at times overwhelms learners and clinicians. Clinicians increasingly report spending more time documenting care processes and interacting with computerized systems than teaching learners (Tierney et al. 2013).

Table 5 highlights not only the benefits and challenges that educational institutions face in using EHR while helping their learners achieve the educational milestones, but also the future directions for research and evaluation (Tierney et al. 2013). If EHR is well utilized, clinical decision support systems can allow for context-specific education, provide opportunities for research/quality improvement projects, and offer a platform for interprofessional interaction. Educational institutions need to implement more strategic planning and training to further integrate EHR into medical education to help learners transition into practice.

Suggested educational approaches to EHR implementation.

EHR can impact effective written communication skills in both positive and negative ways. Academic institutions need to create authentic and controlled EHR simulation environments, where learners can gather information from a simulated patient, be coached on how to best enter information, and then receive feedback on their ability to balance patient

Table 5. Key issues of electronic medical record (EMR) use for accreditation counsel for graduate medical education core competencies

Core Competency	Benefits	Challenges	Future Directions
Medical Knowledge	Point-of-care clinical decision support (CDS) allows for context-relevant education.	Volume of online information may be overwhelming or underused.	Assess impact of CDS on fund of knowledge and identify most useful elements of CDS for learners.
Practice-Based Learning and Improvement	• CDS provides opportunities to teach students and residents best practices. • EMRs offer opportunities in research and quality improvement education.	• CDS may be inappropriate to workflow, and/or may promote alert fatigue. • Functional tools for registry tracking are still nascent.	• Well-planned implementation of CDS may improve teaching opportunities. • Further development of patient-tracking tools will allow greater use in quality improvement.
Patient Care	EMRs can reduce time spent in data gathering and allow for proficient profiling and tracking of trainee clinical experiences and milestones.	EMRs may also introduce workflow inefficiencies and may dull or stunt critical thinking skills.	Evaluate implementation of optimal computerized provider order entry to maximize workflow efficiencies and preserve critical clinical thinking.
Interpersonal and Communication Skills	Learners may spend less time gathering and more time synthesizing clinical data.	Restrictions imposed on use of order entry or charting may limit EMR skill acquisition and documentation proficiency.	Modify documentation systems to promote EMR usage by trainees. Evaluate use of EMR as a tool for mobile, real-time clinical presentations.
Professionalism	Dedicated computer skill teaching can improve patient-provider interaction.	Computer-provider interaction may displace or degrade provider-patient interaction.	Determine how and when EMR-specific patient encounter skills should be introduced and assessed.
Systems-Based Practice	EMRs offer potential for teaching effective integration of a network of care providers.	EMR systems have not reached full maturity to support full multidisciplinary collaboration.	EMR technology needs to advance to fulfill needs of learners to operate effectively in the realm of the patient-centered medical home.

Printed with permission from *Academic Medicine* (Tierney et al. 2013).

engagement with the electronic documentation of the encounter (Pageler et al. 2013). Institutions can make use of the standardized scenarios used in Objective Structured Clinical Exams (OSCE) for evaluation and feedback. Communication to establish relationships between physicians and clinical informatics communities is important to ensure that current EHRs serve medical education, as well as the practice of medicine, while supporting efficient and compassionate care (Delbanco et al. 2012).

At the University of Florida (UF), learners are encouraged to write their own notes without using an already established template during their inpatient rotations; however, most outpatient clinics do use personalized templates that learners may gain access to and use for their notes. Using note templates and copy-and-paste capabilities in charting can dramatically decrease the effectiveness of physician notes as a communication tool (Tierney et al. 2013). Learning to document medical information without relying upon templates is important for developing learners' critical reasoning. On the other hand, if learners lack preclinical EHR training, the process of adapting to a new EHR may be slower and more difficult; it may even interfere with the medical education process, because learners spend more time interacting with a computer instead of the patient. Often the medical documentation itself is the focus of evaluation and feedback by medical educators (Tierney et al. 2013). At UF, learners in the preclinical years have sessions during which they are tasked with documenting history and physical examination in a simulated outpatient setting in our EHR. The students then receive feedback from faculty and the simulated patient on their ability to communicate while using the computer and the quality of the notes. Additionally, during the clinical years, in the course of their inpatient and ambulatory rotations, our students write notes in the EHR in sections designated for student notes, which are reviewed by trained faculty evaluators. Evaluators place particular emphasis on the learner's ability to synthesize the patient encounter in an electronic note correctly and concisely. Learners are also encouraged to use the EHR patient communication tools for after-visit follow-ups and for reviewing test results with their patients. These measures help foster doctor-patient relationships early on in medical training.

An approach to improve EHR transparency (OpenNotes)

The Health Insurance Portability and Accountability Act (HIPAA) provides patients the right to control access and distribution of their medical records. As patients increasingly gain access to the EHR via shared patient-physician portals (OpenNotes) that allow them to read many parts of their medical record, learners will need training to understand the etiquette of direct written patient communication. Educators will need to monitor their learners' electronic communications and ensure that they role-model appropriate use of patient electronic-messaging tools.

Given the complexity and psychosocial ramifications of the medical problems that physicians address daily, it is not surprising to find that physicians have reservations about making their notes available to patients. For example, including a differential diagnosis of malignancy or a concern regarding possible domestic violence in the EHR that a patient can access could lead to a profound breakdown of trust between physician and patient. These scenarios become even more complicated when patients share their chart notes with family members or health surrogates; some patients may even discuss these interactions on social media sites. In the United States, the Communications Decency Act does not hold hosting Web providers accountable for information posted on their sites; thus it is difficult for physicians to protect themselves from defamatory comments or to remove libelous content (Lee et al. 2016). This risk may potentially influence the way that some physicians view the open-note challenge (Lee et al. 2016). Learners may not yet be aware of the impact that note transparency may have in patient-physician relationships or in developing their professional reputation early on in their career. Despite the fear of lawsuits, increasing transparency could conceivably help in patients identifying medical errors and, if used well, could help build trust. If educators can teach the electronic generation of future physicians how to accurately and efficiently document in ways that truly improve patient care, perhaps the phenomenon of practicing "defensive medicine" may come to an end (Lee et al. 2016).

Conceptual Framework: How to Incorporate Social Media into Medical Education

Some researchers have argued that avoidance of social media in medical school curricula may prevent the discovery of positive uses of social media (Chretien and Kind 2014; Fenwick 2014). As medical educators, we should ensure that our learners' online identity molds around their professional identity. They should not need to scramble to change their online information prior to job interviews or need to "hide" their accounts (Chretien and Kind 2014). However, focusing on risk aversion only may not be the best strategy, as it can prevent health care learners and professionals from using social media for beneficial purposes. Chretien and Kind (2014) propose a hierarchy of needs for social media use based on Maslow's psychological theory of a hierarchy of needs, which can be considered as a pyramid where one achieves each level, starting with basic needs prior to reaching the highest level of self-actualization. The foundation of Chretien and Kind's (2014) pyramid is based on *public trust*, which stems from professionalism. While using multiple social networking platforms, busy physicians may not always reflect on privacy violation rules, which may lead to patient distrust. Therefore, it is important to hold physicians accountable for their online behavior. Moving further up the pyramid, Chretien and Kind (2014) describe three main needs to create awareness about physicians' use of social media. Just as food and water are basic needs for human beings, *security* is a basic need in health care professionals' use of social media. This need should be viewed as the stepping stone for medical educators to teach their learners about safe online practices. Once learners achieve this level, the next step is to *reflect* on building an online identity and developing networking connections. The aspirational level of the pyramid is *discovery*, where use of social media enhances knowledge through effective interactions and mentoring relationships with other health professionals; these aim to create a healthier society through innovation and research.

As medical educators, we need to ensure that basic needs of learners are met—that is, they understand the importance of paying attention to online security issues, including patient privacy; they are reflective about the use of social media, and they understand that this technology can be used for discovery and innovation.

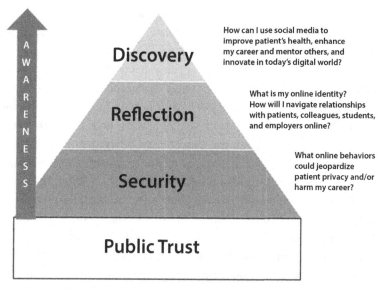

Figure 8. Physicians' social media use as a modified hierarchy of needs. Printed with permission from *Academic Medicine* From K. C. Chretien and T. Kind, Climbing social media in medicine's hierarchy of needs. *Academic Medicine* 89, no. 10 (2014): 1318–1320.

Adapting to Web 2.0 and the Digital Divide

Social media has impacted the way we communicate as a society. The medical profession is not immune from the influence of easily accessible social networking sites such as Facebook, Twitter, and other Web platforms (Chretien and Kind 2013). Medicine is constantly adapting to recent technologies and innovative changes, including social media platforms. In medicine, social media is used in diverse ways and for a variety of reasons. Social media allows for real-time communication and dissemination of innovative ideas between networks of medical professionals. When used for educational purposes, social media enable easy and fast communication among learners and between teachers and learners. For example, students and teachers can pose and answer questions related to classroom assignments; share new insights, such as links to journal articles; and in some instances, communicate with other health care professionals involved in the care of a patient. However, there can be ethical and legal challenges in using social media. In the United States, laws protect patient privacy, and the legal consequences of violating that privacy, discourage sharing sensitive patient information over unsafe communication channels. Additionally, sharing full-text journal articles or educational materials can also violate copyright laws. Consequently, some universities explicitly discourage the use of Facebook for educational purposes, whereas others see it as a suitable alternative means of communication between faculty and their learners (S. H. Jain 2009). We will discuss these issues in depth as they pertain to Facebook and blogs.

In education the concepts of "digital natives" and "digital immigrants" have been used to explain the generational differences between learners and educators. A digital native is a technology user who was born after 1980 into the digital world; a digital immigrant is a technology user, usually born before 1980, who was not born into the digital age and therefore developed their first information literacy in the "print world" (Prensky 2001). Digital natives grew up using various social networking platforms. Web 2.0 represents a second generation of Web-based tools that harness collective intelligence and foster user collaboration. These tools include, but are not limited to: blogs, wikis, media sharing, instant messaging, podcasts, and social networking sites (Sandars and Schroter 2007). It is essential for medical educators to adapt to recent technologies to overcome the "digital divide" (Sandars and Schroter 2007, p. 761). Podcasting is one recent innovation that medical educators are using to provide content to learners "when they want, how they want and where they want" (Boulos et al. 2006, p. 3). Learners, peers, and sometimes faculty use networking platforms to communicate. Such communication may be limited to asking questions related to the logistics of a course, such as, "When is the exam?" or "Where is the workshop being conducted?" or may include instances when educators use Web 2.0 tools to stimulate learning (Boulos et al. 2006). For example, educational users can use Twitter—a "microblogging" site that limits messages to 140 characters—to inform learners of events, share links, and exchange views (Forgie et al. 2013). Some Twitter users also forward succinct published research summaries and notices of upcoming academic meetings. Digital immigrants may adapt to the various Web 2.0 tools, but may find it more difficult to integrate them into their pedagogical practices. Additionally, the generational gap between educators and their learners influences educators' views about the appropriateness of using social media for e-learning, clinical care, and even communicating with peers.

Some physicians use crowdsourcing through online communities, such as Sermo and Doximity, to answer clinical questions and seek expert advice from peers; they join the community after verification of credentials (Chretien and Kind 2013). This form of professional networking is especially helpful for community physicians in private practice, as it reduces isolation while also providing reliable curbside advice.

Facebook

Facebook, one of the largest online free social networking websites, has 1.94 billion monthly active users as of March 31, 2017 (Facebook 2017). The world over, in health professional training and later work environments, students, residents, fellows, attending physicians, and allied health care professionals are connected through Facebook. Often users display their political affiliations, relationship status, and sexual orientation on their online profiles. They may then connect with others with similar interests, and some may use Facebook to organize community action, such as forming political groups to support health care reforms or support groups focusing on specific diseases like diabetes, or rare diseases like cystic fibrosis (S. H. Jain 2009). A study at the University of Florida, Gainesville, reported that 64 percent of medical students use Facebook frequently, versus only 12 percent of residents, with a majority of respondents (83 percent) listing one form of personally identifiable information (Thompson et al. 2008). Further, some patients may send providers Facebook "friend" requests, which some researchers have described as "crossing boundaries" by merging professional and personal lives, leading to various dilemmas (S. H. Jain 2009).

Studies have called for national societies to facilitate the production of guidelines for health care providers and learners to draw upon while posting online (Gorrindo et al. 2008). Many educators, students, and trainees do not use the privacy settings in their Facebook accounts. In fact, Thompson et al. (2008) report that only one-third of trainees made their Facebook accounts private, and some accounts displayed unprofessional material. Although learners are familiar with HIPAA rules and regulations, medical educators and residency program directors continue to encounter unprofessional online conduct. Further complicating the issue, while educators might find content objectionable, learners may not consider the intent of the postings as inappropriate; for example, they may post to reflect on their experiences and seek emotional support from their peers (Wells et al. 2015). At some institutions, students and trainees are explicitly warned about the disconnect between their perceptions and those of program directors or future employers who are likely to search information about candidates on the Internet (S. H. Jain 2009). It is interesting to note that a recent systematic review reported no evidence to support the influence of Facebook on academic performance (Pander et al. 2014).

Researchers also debate the ethical issues arising from health care providers looking up their patients on Facebook. The provider may look up a patient with the intention to help them, but that patient may feel that the doctor has violated his or her personal boundaries, even though the profile information is publicly available. This feeling of violation may in turn impact the doctor-patient relationship. Moreover, there is significant variation in how providers handle sensitive information obtained—for example, information regarding suicidal ideation. Medical professionals have not reached a consensus on appropriate behavior in this area, and research has uncovered little data about the impact on doctor-patient relationship (Jent et al. 2011).

Medical blogs

Maintaining blogs sharing clinical and individual experiences can be therapeutic for educators and learners while at the same time benefiting their colleagues, mentees, and even their patients. However, in a review study of 271 medical blogs written by health care professionals including physicians, nurses, fellows, and residents, 42 percent of the blogs studied described individual patients, with 17 percent of them portraying patients in a negative way (Chretien and Kind 2013). A minority of the blogs even showed photos of patients and endorsed medical products without any conflict-of-interest disclosures. This study stresses the need for medical curriculums to develop norms and standards of medical blog content by medical educators to provide models that promote education while simultaneously reflecting compassion and respect for patients (McGowan et al. 2012). While writing a blog, it is essential to "de-identify" the patient and any unique patient characteristics while also ensuring a respectful tone. It is also important to examine the intent of the writer. On the one hand, a majority of educators accept reflections about the duties of a physician and posts created to stimulate empathy using de-identified information.

On the other hand, educators do not accept posting a patient status update or airing personal frustrations (Chretien and Kind 2013).

Ethical Guidance for Social Media Actions

Doctor-patient communication via social media

Many educators view social media communication, including accepting friend requests by patients, in a negative light. Some have raised concerns have about how to handle situations when "social media friends" ask health-related questions on Facebook. By disclosing personal information on social media sites, physicians risk disrupting the professional boundaries and risk heavy fines and potential criminal charges for unauthorized disclosure of protected health information. Therefore, physicians should avoid accepting friend requests from patients on unsecured, popular third-party sites. Physicians may find it useful to having an open discussion with the patient regarding use of social media (Chretien and Kind 2013). An exception to this avoidance of social media is the use or professional social networking sites where communication with patients remains within the realm of the practice of medicine, and the content of shared information is regulated. However, physicians involved in such sites should exercise caution and respectfully decline to answer direct medical advice questions, as this may have negative legal implications. When individuals seek direct medical advice, physicians should advise them to contact their own physician or make an appointment to discuss their concerns in person (Chretien and Kind 2013). In summary, when directly communicating with patients using social media, physicians should observe the following recommendations: ensure use of a secure encrypted platform; avoid third-party platforms (Facebook, Twitter); inform patients about privacy protections; establish expectations regarding emergencies and physician response time; and have patients agree to terms before use (Chretien and Kind 2013).

There are positive applications of social media in the doctor-patient relationship. Secure portals can provide information to patients, many of whom may otherwise come across unreliable information on the Internet. Physicians are likely to establish better rapport and have more influence if they assist patients with finding trustworthy and easily understandable online medical information. For example, physicians who are knowledgeable about social media applications can guide patients toward appropriate mobile applications for weight loss, smoking cessation, or fitness. Secure patient portals can also enhance the ability of patients and physicians to correspond regarding minor health issues, avoiding unnecessary, time-consuming, and potentially costly office visits.

Evaluating appropriateness of posts

In a survey of U.S. medical schools, 60 percent of the respondent schools reported unprofessional online behavior from their students (Chretien et al. 2009), despite the fact that some of these schools had policies in place pertaining to online behavior. The authors stress the importance of teaching appropriate online behaviors in medical school curriculums as well as familiarizing both students and faculty with HIPAA and Family Educational Rights and Privacy Act (FERPA, 20 U.S.C. § 1232g) policies (Chretien et al. 2009). Another study found that 50 percent of medical students had Facebook profiles, and that medical students on medical mission trips posted unedited photos of patients along with their health information. The authors note the importance of protecting all patients' information, regardless of where health professionals practice (Thompson and Black 2011). Researchers from the University of Michigan used mock medical student Facebook accounts that included different scenarios from their social lives, education, and sexual orientation, to examine the perceptions of medical students, faculty, and the public about the appropriateness of social media posting (A. Jain et al. 2014). The study showed significant differences between these three groups. The faculty group had the most conservative views when it came to the appropriateness of posting, followed by of the general public, and lastly by medical students. The authors attribute the difference in perceptions to the degree of professionalism that the faculty and the general public expects from the medical students and trainees. This study once again emphasizes the need to instill professional online behavior early on in medical education (A. Jain et al. 2014). Another survey noted that 82–84 percent of internal medicine and pediatrics educators felt that it was never or rarely acceptable to become social media friends with their patients (Chretien et al. 2011).

Medical students in our institution (the University of Florida) have dedicated class Facebook pages where they post pertinent updates about upcoming tests and discussions about educational materials, fundraisers, and medical mission trips. The authors of this chapter feel that this form of social media engagement should be encouraged, as it is a great way to encourage group cohesion, socialization, support, and collaboration around the shared medical education experience. On entry to the College of Medicine, students are given guidelines regarding establishing an online professional identity.

The Council of Ethical and Judicial Affairs of the American Medical Association (AMA) has set forth clear recommendations and guidelines about professionalism in the use of social media, which all medical students and other medical professionals can easily access. It is important to make learners aware of these important guidelines early on in their training to avoid unintended consequences, which may negatively impact their future professional careers (AMA 2010). In its position paper on professionalism in the era of Web 2.0, the American College of Physicians encourages reflection before posting online on the ethical crux of online behavior, stating that "consideration should be given to how patients and the public would perceive the material" (Farnan et al. 2013, p. 5). Additionally, the AMA advises physicians to report unprofessional online content to the relevant authorities (AMA 2010).

Physician online ratings

Physicians frequently encounter patients who, prior to establishing care, have researched the physicians on the Internet. Often, health professionals encourage patient reviews of their health care experiences on various websites to obtain feedback and improve on health care delivery. Researchers have debated the usefulness of such feedback, as most patients give their physicians a favorable rating (Kadry et al. 2011). The surveys on feedback websites often contain a comprehensive list of many elements related to patient experience, from the office environment and staff courtesy to physician timeliness, ability to make a correct diagnosis, care, and compassion. Notably, the AMA has not approved the development of physician-rating websites because, since the reviewers are anonymous, the physicians' responses may be hampered by patient privacy issues, resulting in negative reviews (Lagu et al. 2010). Furthermore, some have expressed concern that patients who rate their physicians on these websites had a one-time negative experience that does not represent the many other patients cared for by that specific physician. Such events could potentially result in defamation of physicians and undue emotional and psychological stress for physicians (Strech 2011). Despite concerns, physician-rating websites continue to grow, and remain a source of information for many patients. A study evaluating 190 reviews of 81 physicians found 88 percent positive ratings, 6 percent negative ratings, and 6 percent neutral ratings (Lagu et al. 2010). The study did not report a difference between generalists and subspecialty physicians. Interestingly, the authors also identified a subset of reviews posted by the physicians themselves. These reviews contained information about their education, training, and services offered, and were easily distinguishable from patient postings (Lagu et al. 2010). In a survey of patients, 59 percent responded that physician rating sites were "somewhat important" or "very important" (Kadry et al. 2011). As rating scales grow, physicians, educators, and learners must not practice defensive medicine to avoid getting a "bad grade" from their patients (Sabin 2013, p. 935). Most recent health care initiatives, like those set forth by large governmental organizations such as Medicare in the United States, evaluate physicians and hospitals based on performance measures and adherence to specific clinical guidelines; at this time, however, they do not allow patients to rate the provider (Lagu et al. 2010).

Final Thoughts

As EHR and social media have become important aspects of all facets of health care, the need for collaboration among groups of educators, learners, clinicians, health care organizations, lawmakers, and patients has become even more apparent. More studies are required to specifically address the EHR training process of future physicians (medical students and residents). The scenarios at the start of the chapter reflect current dilemmas faced by educators. The first brings to light how learners and attending physicians rely on information stored in the EHR. The learners often meet an "i-patient"—that is, the patient's chart serves as a surrogate for the patient (Wear et al. 2015). Educators therefore not only face the challenge of ensuring that essential history taking and communication skills are fulfilled, but also need to deliberately construct space in the curriculum for such encounters. The second scenario portrays the importance of educating learners about ethics and privacy issues related to online posts, whereas the third scenario shows how learners and physicians have to be sensitized to ensure that their well-meaning posts do not contain potential patient identifiers. In this case, by looking up the oncologist's admitting privileges, a reader of her blog could discern which hospital the patient is admitted in and, in a small community, may be able to identify the patient based on the description of the family, which would likely constitute a HIPAA violation.

Questions for Future Research

What is the impact of OpenNotes on the doctor-patient relationship?

What is the effectiveness of potential mechanisms to reduce the impact of EHR on the potential for physician burnout?

Does the EHR actually encourage and increase the likelihood of interprofessional collaboration in quality and patient safety?

Which curricula are most effective in engendering a culture of online professionalism?

What impact does social media have on the formation of learners' professional identity?

References

American Medical Association (AMA). (2010). AMA policy: Professionalism in the use of social media. Retrieved June 27, 2012, from: http://www.ama-assn.org/ama/pub/meeting/professionalism-social-media.shtml.

Boulos, M. N., Maramba, I., and Wheeler, S. (2006). Wikis, blogs and podcasts: A new generation of Web-based tools for virtual collaborative clinical practice and education. *BMC Medical Education* 6(1): 41. doi: 10.1186/1472-6920-6-41.

Chretien, K. C., Farnan, J. M., Greysen, S. R., and Kind, T. (2011). To friend or not to friend? Social networking and faculty perceptions of online professionalism. *Academic Medicine* 86(12): 1545–1550. doi: 10.1097/acm.0b013e3182356128.

Chretien, K. C., Greysen, S. R., Chretien, J., and Kind, T. (2009). Online posting of unprofessional content by medical students. *JAMA* 302(12): 1309–1315. doi: 10.1001/jama.2009.1387.

Chretien, K. C., and Kind, T. (2013). Social media and clinical care: Ethical, professional, and social implications. *Circulation* 127(13): 1413–1421. doi: 10.1161/circulationaha.112.128017.

Chretien, K. C., and Kind, T. (2014). Climbing social media in medicine's hierarchy of needs. *Academic Medicine* 89(10): 1318–1320. doi: 10.1097/acm.0000000000000430.

Delbanco, T., Walker, J., Bell, S. K., Darer, J. D., Elmore, J. G., Farag, N., . . . Leveille, S. G. (2012). Inviting patients to read their doctors' notes: A quasi-experimental study and a look ahead. *Annals of Internal Medicine* 157(7): 461–470. doi: 10.7326/0003-4819-157-7-201210020-00002.

Facebook. (2017). Company info. Retrieved July 1, 2017, from https://newsroom.fb.com/company-info/.

Farnan, J. M., Snyder Sulmasy, L., Worster, B. K., Chaudhry, H. J., Rhyne, J. A., Arora, V. M., . . . Federation of State Medical Boards Special Committee on Ethics and Professionalism. (2013). Online medical professionalism: Patient and public relationships: Policy statement from the American College of Physicians and the Federation of State Medical Boards. *Annals of Internal Medicine* 158(8): 620–627. doi: 10.7326/0003-4819-158-8-201304160-00100.

Fenwick, T. (2014). Social media and medical professionalism: Rethinking the debate and the way forward. *Academic Medicine* 89(10): 1331–1334. doi: 10.1097/acm.0000000000000436.

Forgie, S. E., Duff, J. P., and Ross, S. (2013). Twelve tips for using Twitter as a learning tool in medical education. *Medical Teacher* 35(1): 8–14. doi: 10.3109/0142159x.2012.746448.

Gorrindo, T., Gorrindo, P. C., and Groves, J. E. (2008). Intersection of online social networking with medical professionalism: Can medicine police the Facebook boom? *Journal of General Internal Medicine* 23(12): 2155–2155. doi: 10.1007/s11606-008-0810-y.

Jain, A., Petty, E. M., Jaber, R. M., Tackett, S., Purkiss, J., Fitzgerald, J., and White, C. (2014). What is appropriate to post on social media? Ratings from students, faculty members and the public. *Medical Education* 48(2): 157–169. doi: 10.1111/medu.12282.

Jain, S. H. (2009). Practicing edicine in the age of Facebook. *New England Journal of Medicine* 361(7): 649–651. doi: 10.1056/nejmp0901277.

Jent, J. F., Eaton, C. K., Merrick, M. T., Englebert, N. E., Dandes, S. K., Chapman, A. V., and Hershorin, E. R. (2011). The decision to access patient information from a social media site: What would you do? *Journal of Adolescent Health* 49(4): 414–420. doi: 10.1016/j.jadohealth.2011.02.004.

Kadry, B., Chu, L. F., Kadry, B., Gammas, D., and Macario, A. (2011). Analysis of 4999 online physician ratings indicates that most patients give physicians a favorable rating. *Journal of Medical Internet Research* 13(4). doi: 10.2196/jmir.1960.

Lagu, T., Hannon, N. S., Rothberg, M. B., and Lindenauer, P. K. (2010). Patients' evaluations of health care providers in the era of social networking: An analysis of physician-rating websites. *Journal of General Internal Medicine* 25(9): 942–946. doi: 10.1007/s11606-010-1383-0.

Lee, B. S., Walker, J., Delbanco, T., and Elmore, J. G. (2016). Transparent electronic health records and lagging laws. *Annals of Internal Medicine* 165(3): 219–220. doi: 10.7326/m15-2827.

McGowan, B. S., Wasko, M., Vartabedian, B. S., Miller, R. S., Freiherr, D. D., and Abdolrasulnia, M. (2012). Understanding the factors that influence the adoption and meaningful use of social media by physicians to share medical information. *Journal of Medical Internet Research* 14(5): e117. doi: 10.2196/jmir.2138.

Mintz, M., Narvarte, H. J., O'Brien, K. E., Papp, K. K., Thomas, M., and Durning, S. J. (2009). Use of electronic medical records by physicians and students in academic internal medicine settings. *Academic Medicine* 84(12): 1698–1704. doi: 10.1097/ acm.0b013e3181bf9d45.

Pageler, N. M., Friedman, C. P., and Longhurst, C. A. (2013). Refocusing medical education in the EMR era. *JAMA* 310(21): 2249–2250. doi: 10.1001/jama.2013.282326.

Pander, T., Pinilla, S., Dimitriadis, K., and Fischer, M. R. (2014). The use of Facebook in medical education—A literature review. *GMS Zeitschrift Fur Medizinische Ausbildung* 31(3): Doc33. doi: 10.3205/zma000925.

Prensky, M. (2001). Digital natives, digital immigrants. *On the Horizon* 9(5): 1–6. doi: 10.1108/10748120110424816.

Sabin, J. E. (2013). Physician-rating websites. *Virtual Mentor* 15(11): 932–936. doi: 10.1001/ virtualmentor.2013.15.11.ecas2-1311.

Sandars, J., and Schroter, S. (2007). Web 2.0 technologies for undergraduate and postgraduate medical education: An online survey. *Postgraduate Medical Journal* 83(986): 759–762. doi: 10.1136/pgmj.2007.063123.

Strech, D. (2011). Ethical principles for physician rating sites. *Journal of Medical Internet Research* 13(4): e113. doi: 10.2196/jmir.1899.

Thompson, L. A., and Black, E. W. (2011). Nonclinical use of online social networking sites: New and old challenges to medical professionalism. *Journal of Clinical Ethics* 22(2): 179–182.

Thompson, L. A., Dawson, K., Ferdig, R., Black, E. W., Boyer, J., Coutts, J., and Black, N. P. (2008). The intersection of online social networking with medical professionalism. *Journal of General Internal Medicine* 23(7): 954–957. doi: 10.1007/s11606-008-0538-8.

Tierney, M. J., Pageler, N. M., Kahana, M., Pantaleoni, J. L., and Longhurst, C. A. (2013, 06). Medical education in the electronic medical record (EMR) era. *Academic Medicine* 88(6): 748–752. doi: 10.1097/acm.0b013e3182905ceb.

Wear, D., Zarconi, J., Kumagai, A., and Cole-Kelly, K. (2015). Slow medical education. *Academic Medicine* 90(3): 289–293. doi: 10.1097/acm.0000000000000581.

Wells, D. M., Lehavot, K., and Isaac, M. L. (2015). Sounding off on social media. *Academic Medicine* 90(8): 1015–1019. doi: 10.1097/acm.0000000000000668.

12

Introspection about Role Modeling

JUAN GUARDERAS, MAUREEN NOVAK, AND CAROLYN STALVEY[1]

Ut sementem feceris ita metes—As you sow, so shall you reap.
Cicero

We discuss how role modeling encompasses clinical, teaching, and personal qualities. Positive and negative attributes of role models are described, and we introduce readers to the concept of "role modeling consciousness." In addition, the chapter provides strategies for educators seeking to improve their role-modeling skills.

Objectives

Describe the different facets of role modeling in academic medicine.
Understand the role-model continuum.
Describe a conceptual framework for role modeling.

At the end of a very busy clinic, Dr. Patel asks Stavros to reflect on what he saw her do as an attending during the clinic. The student smiles and says, "I noticed that despite Mrs. Smith's obvious poor hygiene, you treated her the same as you did the lady before wearing all that bling!"

As we were completing our walking rounds on our team's patients, the intern stopped right outside the door of the patient's room and said, "She is back! LJ is here again. . . ." The senior resident and other interns groaned. The attending smiled and said, "Oh come on, it can't be that bad, tell me. . . ." Turns out she was known to have lupus with end-stage renal disease and was a "very difficult patient."

---

1   Juan Guarderas, M.D., University of Florida College of Medicine, Gainesville, FL.
     Maureen Novak, M.D., University of Florida College of Medicine, Gainesville, FL.
     Carolyn Stalvey, M.D., University of Florida College of Medicine, Gainesville, FL.

I was in an exam room with Dr. Casey, the Hematology-Oncology attending, and after informing Ms. Hardy that her metastatic breast cancer was worse—now stage four—he proceeded to discuss the plan for further chemotherapy, without pausing to address her emotions or ask her for her thoughts. And then that was it. . . . He walked out of the exam room!

In 1910 Abraham Flexner recognized the importance of the role teachers play in the complex process of developing a competent physician, during which medical novices need the opportunity to practice skills under the guidance of an experienced teacher (Flexner 1910). The American sociologist Robert Merton (1910–2003) first coined the term "role model" in a study on the socialization of medical students (Calhoun 2010). Since then, role modeling has been highlighted in medical education literature as a phenomenon that influences the professional development and career choices of students (Cruess et al. 2008; Passi et al. 2013; Wright and Carrese 2002). While *Merriam-Webster* defines a role model as "a person whose behavior in a particular role is imitated by others" (*Merriam-Webster OnLine* n.d., s.v. "role model"), Burgess et al. (2015a) describe role modeling in medical education as a process during which faculty members demonstrate clinical skills, model and articulate expertise, share their thought processes, and manifest positive professional characteristics. Boerebach et al. (2012) also describe role modeling as "an overarching activity that encompasses everything faculty do in their being and acting as professionals" (p. 1) and is at the "heart of character formation" (Cruess et al. 2008, p. 718).

The terms apprenticeship, role modeling, and mentoring are often used interchangeably, but they have different pedagogical meaning. *Merriam-Webster* defines an apprentice as a person who learns a job or skill by working for a fixed period for someone who is very good at that job (*Merriam-Webster Online* n.d., s.v. "apprentice"). In contrast, a role model is a person whom the learner admires, aspires to be like, and whose behavior the learner tries to imitate (Swick et al. 1999). Mentors, however, are senior members of a group who intentionally encourage and support junior colleagues in their careers (Ramani et al. 2006). Some institutions have structured mentoring programs with training opportunities or resources for both mentors and mentees. Unlike mentorship, being a role model is generally serendipitous, with no associated training (Paice et al. 2002). Role modeling can be less intentional and often subliminal, more informal, and more episodic than mentoring (Kenny et al. 2003). Mentors may or may not be a role model for their learners, depending on the relationship or structure of the program. Table 6 summarizes these definitions and provides newer definitions of these terms based on available literature.

Table 6. Definition of terms

Term	Old Definition	New Definition	Examples
Apprentice/ ship	"One who is learning by practical experience under skilled workers a trade, art, or calling" (*Merriam-Webster OnLine* n.d., "apprentice")	Apprenticeship is defined as "legitimate peripheral participation" (Dornan 2005, p. 95) while developing a professional identity by socializing into a community of professional learning and practice (Bleakley 2002; Dornan 2005)	The preregistration house officers in the UK (Bleakley 2002)
Role model/ modeling	Role models demonstrate clinical skills, model and articulate expertise thought processes, and manifest positive professional characteristics (Irby 1986; Jochemsen-van der Leeuw et al. 2013)	Role modeling is the conscious and subconscious process by default role models that is highly dependent on the attributes of role models and the judgments made by the modellee (person influenced by the modeling process) through reflection and apperception (Jochemsen-van der Leeuw et al. 2013)	Any faculty and other allied health professional in contact with learners
Mentor/ship	Mentor is actively engaged in an explicit two-way relationship with the junior colleague—a relationship that evolves and develops over time and can be terminated by either party (Ramani et al. 2006; Rose et al. 2005; Sachdeva 1996)	Mentoring can be formal (structured program) or informal and can convey explicit academic knowledge, enhance implicit knowledge about professionalism through role modeling, and can provide emotional support to mentees, while helping them in attaining success (Ramani et al. 2006; Rose et al. 2005)	Formal institutional mentoring programs or informal mentorship provided

Compiled by authors.

Attributes of Role Models

Researchers have identified various characteristics of role modeling and clustered them into three attributes: *clinical, teaching,* and *personal quali-ties* (Cruess et al. 2008; Wright and Carrese, 2002). In the *clinical attri-butes* category, good role modeling demonstrates a patient-centered ap-proach with strong clinical skills, humanistic behavior, empathy, respect, and compassion (Althouse et al. 1999; Elzubeir and Rizk 2001; Passi et al. 2013). Regarding *teaching attributes,* the best role models provide a large number of teaching activities and patient interactions (Wright et al. 1997). While acknowledging the importance of a patient-centered approach, students note that faculty with ideal attributes of a role model demon-strate excellence in teaching skills by providing constructive learning en-vironments and catering to the learning needs of students (Burgess et al. 2015b). Enhancing faculty's overall teaching performance may therefore improve role modeling (Boerebach et al. 2012). The *personal attributes* researchers associate with good role modeling include leadership skills, enthusiasm, dedication, interpersonal skills, honesty, respect for interpro-fessional staff, passion, commitment to excellence, and ability to inspire (Burgess et al. 2015a, p. 2; Swanwick 2005; Wright and Carrese 2001). In a survey assessing the qualities of a good role model, students did not give significant weight to publications, grants, seniority and leadership, physi-cal appearance, and interests outside of medicine (Elzubeir and Rizk 2001; Paice et al. 2002). In a systematic review of the literature, Jochemsen-van der Leeuw et al. (2013) identify an extensive list of attributes describing positive and negative role models, which are summarized in Table 7.

The current literature mostly focuses on the positive aspects of role modeling (Kenny et al. 2003; Wright et al. 1998), but recent debates high-light the potential for role modeling to have negative impacts as well as positive ones (Paice et al. 2002). For example, researchers note that stu-dents learn by observing role models and then imitating those behaviors (Crosby 2000). This imitation may initially help students adapt to the clinical environment, but, if sustained, can result in undesirable behaviors such as doctor-centered interviewing or discrimination between insured and uninsured patients (Benbassat 2014). Students report that it is not uncommon for faculty to make cynical comments about the profession, which in turn has a negative impact on students' career choices (Kenny et al. 2003; Wear et al. 2009). When students witness derogatory humor in

Table 7. Summary of positive and negative attributes of role models

Patient Care Qualities	Teaching Qualities	Personal Qualities
POSITIVE ATTRIBUTES		
• Is competent	• Employs a humanistic style of teaching	• Is patient
• Has up-to-date knowledge of the field	• Establishes rapport with learners	• Has self-confidence
• Is experienced	• Tailors teaching to learners' needs	• Has self-esteem
• Is committed to excellence and growth	• Creates a safe learning environment	• Displays honesty and integrity
• Has effective diagnostic and therapeutic skills	• Gives learners the autonomy to make independent decisions	• Is easy to work with and cooperative
• Demonstrates sound clinical reasoning	• Teaches trainees about the psychological aspects of medicine and the importance of the doctor-patient relationship	• Shows humility and humanism
• Is compassionate, caring, engaging	• Adopts a positive attitude toward trainees	• Has leadership ability
• Is empathic to patients	• Shows enthusiasm for teaching	
• Is able to build a personal connection with patients	• Makes himself or herself available for trainees	
• Is dedicated to the quality of patient care	• Is accessible for questions	
• Centers the care he or she provides on the patient rather than the illness	• Stimulates critical thinking	
• Communicates well with patients and their relatives	• Makes learning exciting and is inspirational	
• Shows respect to patients	• Is aware of the importance of his or her role-model status for medical education and acts as a dedicated and active role model, encouraging the trainee to adopt similar behavior	
• Has a humanistic attitude toward patients		
• Educates and fully informs patients		
• Respects and gives recognition to others, resulting in positive interactions with other health care workers		
• Exhibits a high degree of professionalism		
• Assumes responsibility in difficult clinical situations		
• Is able to cope with adversity		
• Demonstrates enthusiasm for work and enjoys the job		
• Displays satisfaction with his or her chosen specialty		
NEGATIVE ATTRIBUTES		
• Is uncaring and communicates poorly with patients	• Teaches the trainee the wrong thing to do and the wrong way to behave	• Is cynical
• Adopts an uncooperative attitude toward health care workers	• Gives poor support to learners	• Has a sexist attitude
• Displays unprofessional attitudes and unethical behavior	• Rarely provides feedback to trainees	• Is impatient, inflexible, and overly opinionated
• Does not have up-to-date knowledge of the field	• Practices a sink-or-swim approach from the outset	• May nitpick and be harsh, unfair, or self-serving
	• Is disinterested and has difficulty remembering names and faces	• May lack self-confidence or leadership skills
		• May be quiet and reserved or overextended

Content of this table is produced with permission from *Academic Medicine* (Jochemsen-van der Leeuw et al. 2013).

clinical settings, they are disappointed by their role models and develop a sense of powerlessness and conflict in their clerkships (Wear et al. 2009). When physicians display a lack of empathy or insensitivity to patients, students often feel uncomfortable and perceive the physicians as negative role models (Burgess et al. 2015a, p. 3). Conversely, positive role models demonstrate respect for the patient both in and out of the patient's room. Positive role models also exhibit conscientiousness and dutifulness, and they strive for excellence (Hojat et al. 1999).

Specific examples of behavior that good role models exhibit include: establishing close doctor-patient relationships, viewing the patient as a whole, sitting or kneeling at the bedside to be at the patient's level, and showing empathy toward patients (Ambrozy et al. 1997; Burgess et al. 2015a, p. 3; Burgess et al. 2015b, p. 2; Egnew and Wilson 2011). Positive role models devote more time to demonstrating the importance of the doctor-patient relationship and the psychosocial aspects of medical care (Burgess et al. 2015a, p. 3).

Studies have also documented that being honest with the learner regarding the elements of diagnostic uncertainty is an important characteristic of a good role model (Egnew and Wilson 2011). Sharing strategies for handling the diagnostic and therapeutic uncertainty of patient care can normalize any similar feelings the learners may have. As expected, role models who regularly consult the medical literature are more highly rated, as they validate the notion of uncertainty in medicine (Cruess et al. 2008). Highly ranked role models also accept students' mistakes and provide reassurance to students that it is acceptable to be unsure (Althouse et al. 1999).

Students note a disassociation between what they had been taught in the classroom and the real clinical world. The pressures of the health care system limit the time spent with patients. Students feel that they adopt the poor behaviors of role models by "cutting off patients or ignoring patient's emotions" in the interest of time (Egnew and Wilson 2011, p. 102). This "hidden curriculum," which includes unofficial, unintended lessons, can lead to subliminal teaching (Hafferty 1998; Wright et al. 1997). Therefore, how faculty balance the pressures of modern clinical medicine can offer teachable moments. When medical students in Canada were asked to what extent their teachers behaved as humanistic caregivers, 25 percent of second-year students and 40 percent of senior students noted that the faculty did not behave as humanistic caregivers or good role models (Maheux et al. 2000). Notably, by exhibiting reflection and self-awareness, role models may help avoid their own burnout (Cruess et al. 2008).

Learners exposed to a general internist attending have been documented to be more likely to choose a primary care field (Henderson et al. 1996). Unfortunately, students often encounter their role models in the final year of medical school, which is when they make decisions about their specialty choices (Basco and Reigart 2001). As they go through medical training, students often struggle to develop a professional identity in the complex learning environment (Byszewski et al. 2012). Settings with continuity of care and continuity of teaching establish trust between teacher and student that parallels the doctor-patient relationships and can be helpful for the students (Branch et al. 2001).

Role Modeling Consciousness

Role modeling occurs from the first encounter the learner has with the teacher. Therefore, the teacher must realize that all his or her actions are being observed, and must be self-aware and mindful (Egnew and Wilson 2011). Wright and Carrese (2002) term this self-awareness "role modeling consciousness." In their study, faculty who have been identified by several residents as excellent role models note that they "consciously think about being a role model" and are "aware that medical learners are watching" (p. 641). These faculty purposely try to "set the right tone" and make a "conscious effort to role model professionalism and humanism" (Wright and Carrese 2002, p. 641). This behavior is similar to the Hawthorne Effect, which states that people behave differently when they know they are being observed (Jones 1992).

In contrast to the ideal education environment that Flexner proposed, the post-Flexner era is marked by clinical practice that is subspecialized rather than holistic and integrated, and by educational efforts that are often limited by time and competing priorities rather than a solely learner-centered approach. Duty hours and technology issues exert pressure on the learners that further compromises the patient-centered approach (Dornan 2005). Creating an effective relationship between the faculty and the learner while juggling these demands can improve the educational process, which includes gaining knowledge, seeing it applied, and developing the learner's career (Dimitriadis et al. 2012).

Conceptual Framework

Clinician-educators are aware of the importance of role modeling, but when asked how they role-model, they struggle with providing examples (Côté and Leclère 2000). In order to enhance their ability to consciously act as role models, educators require training. Such training should be provided at an individual as well as institutional level. Transformative training experiences can include holding faculty development sessions to create the awareness of being a role model; encouraging faculty to consciously role-model a positive attitude; reflecting and debriefing students; and making a conscious effort to articulate what they are modeling (Cruess et al. 2008). Students highly value faculty role models who try to make implicit messages explicit by articulating relationships and by describing their own interpersonal struggles (Egnew and Wilson 2011). Exemplary role modeling comprises "role modeling consciousness" which, as described earlier, is an awareness of one's role while interacting with trainees (Wright and Carrese 2002). This practice of reflecting on what has been modeled raises awareness about behaviors and can help break the silence for faculty and students (Kenny et al. 2003).

Figure 9 describes the complex process of role modeling, which includes awareness and reflection about conscious behaviors, while processing unconscious behaviors into principles and action (Paice et al. 2002).

According to Bandura's (1989) social learning theory, learning is a social process in which the learner observes the teacher while moving through four processes: attention, retention, reproduction (imitation), and motivation. As learners go through these processes, it is important that they be able to differentiate between positive and negative role modeling. Figure 10 presents the mental process by which students assimilate a new experience and evaluate it in view of past experiences, leading to transformative thought. This process is called apperception and can be used by learners before deciding to imitate behavior (Jochemsen-van der Leeuw et al. 2013).

The scenarios at the start of the chapter highlight situations where educators display positive and negative attributes of role modeling, which influence learners. The student with Dr. Patel noted that she treated the patient with poor personal hygiene no differently from other patients. This observation will likely impact how the student behaves toward patients in the future. In contrast, in the second scenario, when the attending smiles

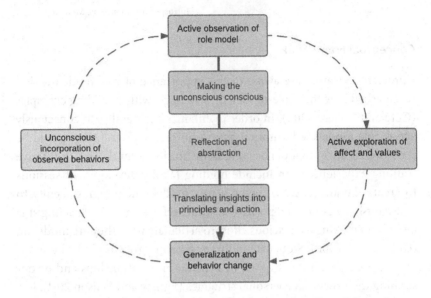

Figure 9. The process of role modeling. Printed with permission. From E. Paice, S. Heard, and F. Moss, "How important are role models in making good doctors?" *BMJ* (Clinical Research Ed.) 325, 7366 (2002): 707–710.

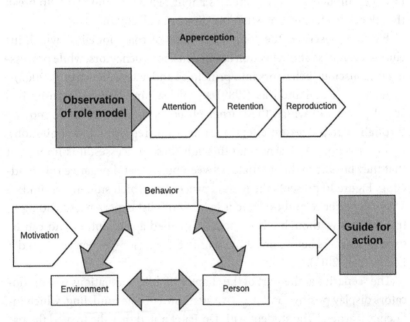

Figure 10. Apperception process. Printed with permission. From H. G. Jochemsen-van der Leeuw, N. van Dijk, F. S. van Etten-Jamaludin, and M. Wieringa-de Waard, "The attributes of the clinical trainer as a role model: A systematic review," *Academic Medicine: Journal of the Association of American Medical Colleges* 88, no. 1 (2013): 26–34.

and comments that the situation cannot be "that bad," she was joined in unprofessional behavior by the junior team members. Additionally, she has role-modeled this behavior to students, who may imitate the same behavior. The third scenario demonstrates how busy clinicians may not pause to address patient emotions and concerns. Students and trainees witnessing such dismissive and abrupt behavior may experience cognitive dissonance, in that such behavior is in sharp contrast to what they are taught in medical school. The dissonance experienced can in turn result in distress and burnout among learners.

Final Thoughts

One hundred years post-Flexner, medical education still struggles with problems related to the hidden curriculum and impact of role modeling (Cooke et al. 2006). Although there have been pedagogical advances, institutions and faculty involved in curriculum design need to pay attention to help learners adapt to the circumstances of the current practice of medicine. Challenges to care and education include keeping up-to-date with advances in diagnosis and therapy as well as required information technology skills. The medical, legal, and socioeconomic challenges faced in patient care influence many decisions in daily practice. Role modeling and the relationship between the faculty member and the learner are even more important in this day and age and have significant untapped potential. Faculty development to create awareness of the subconscious process of role modeling (Figure 9) is essential to help them understand how to make the implicit explicit. Sessions with learners are important too, to help them understand how to reflect on the behaviors of role models and avoid imitation of negative behaviors. Both educators and students need to understand that being a role model is an ideal to be pursued (Cruess et al. 2008). Perfection is not possible all the time, but it is a goal to strive for. Role models are an important part of the educational process, and educators must learn to navigate these influences while maintaining educational goals. Cruess et al. (2008) provide a summary of strategies for individuals to improve role modeling,which are summarized below:

Be aware of being a role model.
Demonstrate clinical competence.
Protect time for teaching.

Show a positive attitude for what you do.
Implement a student-centered approach to teaching.
Facilitate reflection on clinical experiences and what has been modeled.
Encourage dialogue with colleagues.
Engage in pertinent staff development.
Work to improve the institutional culture.
Whenever possible, be explicit about what you are modeling.

When faculty are overworked and lack support for teaching activities, institutional culture directly impacts role modeling (Hafferty 1998). Strategies to influence institutional culture include increasing awareness, pointing out deficiencies, and proposing remedial actions (Cruess et al. 2008).

The groundwork that has been laid by explicit instruction in professionalism, combined with effective role modeling and attention to the hidden curriculum of the practice environment, can support the development of a comprehensive and sophisticated understanding of professional education. (Cooke et al. 2006)

Issues for Future Research

Specific strategies to develop faculty and improve role modeling.
Development of evaluation tools for assessing the awareness of role modeling and competence as a role model.
Evaluation of the effect of role modeling by gender, ethnicity, and generation.
Per Jochemsen-van der Leeuw et al. (2013), use of the positive and negative attributes described in Table 7 to develop a tool that trainees can use to evaluate faculty.
Creation of training sessions that use apperception to identify traits of role models before imitating them.
The impact of institutional actions to promote a culture that fosters and rewards positive role modeling (Dewey et al. 2005). Strategically identifying such educators could help create a cadre of faculty who serve as effective role models.

References

Althouse, L. A., Stritter, F. T., and Steiner, B. D. (1999). Attitudes and approaches of influential role models in clinical education. *Advances in Health Sciences Education* 4(2): 111–122. doi: 10.1023/a:1009768526142.

Ambrozy, D. M., Irby, D. M., Bowen, J. L., Burack, J. H., Carline, J. D., and Stritter, F. T. (1997). Role models' perceptions of themselves and their influence on students' specialty choices. *Academic Medicine* 72(12): 1119–21. doi: 10.1097/00001888-199712000-00028.

Bandura, A. (1989). Social cognitive theory. In Vasta, R. (ed.): *Annals of child development: Six theories of child development* (vol. 6). Greenwich, CT: JAI Press.

Basco, W. T., and Reigart, J. R. (2001). When do medical students identify career-influencing physician role models? *Academic Medicine* 76(4): 380–382. doi: 10.1097/00001888-200104000-00017.

Benbassat, J. (2014). Role modeling in medical education: The importance of a reflective imitation. *Academic Medicine* 89(4): 550–554. doi: 10.1097/acm.0000000000000189.

Bleakley, A. (2002). Pre-registration house officers and ward-based learning: A "new apprenticeship" model. *Medical Education* 36(1): 9–15. doi: 10.1046/j.1365-2923.2002.01128.x.

Boerebach, B. C., Lombarts, K. M., Keijzer, C., Heineman, M. J., and Arah, O. A. (2012). The teacher, the physician and the person: How faculty's teaching performance influences their role modelling. *PLoS ONE, 7*(3): e32089. doi: 10.1371/journal.pone.0032089.

Branch, W. T. Jr., Kern, D., Haidet, P., Weissmann, P., Gracey, C. F. Mitchell, G., and Inui, T. (2001). Teaching the human dimensions of care in clinical settings. *JAMA* 286(9): 1067–1074. doi: 10.1001/jama.286.9.1067.

Burgess, A., Goulston, K., and Oates, K. (2015a. Role modelling of clinical tutors: A focus group study among medical students. *BMC Medical Education* 15(1). doi: 10.1186/s12909-015-0303-8.

Burgess, A., Oates, K., and Goulston, K. (2015b). Role modelling in medical education: The importance of teaching skills. *Clinical Teacher* 13(2): 134–137. doi: 10.1111/tct.12397.

Byszewski, A., Hendelman, W., McGuinty, C., and Moineau, G. (2012). Wanted: Role models—medical students' perceptions of professionalism. *BMC Medical Education* 12(1). doi: 10.1186/1472-6920-12-115.

Calhoun, C. J. (2010). In Calhoun, C. J. (ed.), *Robert K. Merton: Sociology of science and sociology as science*. New York: Columbia University Press.

Cooke, M., Irby, D. M., Sullivan, W., and Ludmerer, K. M. (2006). American medical education 100 years after the Flexner Report. *New England Journal of Medicine* 355(13): 1339–1344. doi: 10.1056/nejmra055445.

Côté, L., and Leclère, H. (2000). How clinical teachers perceive the doctor—Patient relationship and themselves as role models. *Academic Medicine* 75(11): 1117–1124. doi: 10.1097/00001888-200011000-00020.

Crosby, R. H. (2000). AMEE Guide no. 20: The good teacher is more than a lecturer—the twelve roles of the teacher. *Medical Teacher* 22(4): 334–347. doi: 10.1080/014215900409429.

Cruess, S. R., Cruess, R. L., and Steinert, Y. (2008). Role modelling—making the most of a powerful teaching strategy. *BMJ* 336(7646): 718–721. doi: 10.1136/bmj.39503.757847. be.

Dewey, C. M., Friedland, J. A., Richards, B. F., Lamki, N., and Kirkland, R. T. (2005). The emergence of academies of educational excellence: A survey of U.S. medical schools. *Academic Medicine* 80(4): 358–365. doi: 10.1097/00001888-200504000-00012.

Dimitriadis, K., von der Borch, P. V., Störmann, S., Meinel, F. G., Moder, S., Reincke, M., and Fischer, M. R. (2012). Characteristics of mentoring relationships formed by medical students and faculty. *Medical Education Online* 17(1): 17242. doi: 10.3402/meo.v17i0.17242.

Dornan, T. (2005). Osler, Flexner, apprenticeship and "the new medical education." *Journal of the Royal Society of Medicine* 98(3): 91–95. doi: 10.1258/jrsm.98.3.91.

Egnew, T. R., and Wilson, H. J. (2011). Role modeling the doctor-patient relationship in the clinical curriculum. *Family Medicine* 43(2): 99–105.

Elzubeir, M. A., and Rizk, D. E. (2001). Identifying characteristics that students, interns and residents look for in their role models. *Medical Education* 35(3): 272–277. doi: 10.1111/j.1365-2923.2001.00870.x.

Flexner, A. (1910). *Medical education in the United States and Canada: A report to the Carnegie Foundation for the Advancement of Teaching.* Boston, MA: Updyke.

Hafferty, F. W. (1998). Beyond curriculum reform: Confronting medicine's hidden curriculum. *Academic Medicine* 73(4): 403–407. doi: 10.1097/00001888-199804000-00013.

Henderson, M. C., Hunt, D. K., and Williams, J. W., Jr. (1996). General internists influence students to choose primary care careers: The power of role modeling. *American Journal of Medicine* 101(6): 648–653. doi: 10.1016/s0002-9343(96)00334-8.

Hojat, M., Nasca, T. J., Magee, M., Feeney, K., Pascual, R., Urbano, F., and Gonnella, J. S. (1999). A comparison of the personality profiles of internal medicine residents, physician role models, and the general population. *Academic Medicine* 74(12): 1327–1333. doi: 10.1097/00001888-199912000-00017.

Irby, D. M. (1986). Clinical teaching and the clinical teacher. *Academic Medicine* 61(9): 35–45. doi: 10.1097/00001888-198609000-00005.

Jochemsen-van der Leeuw, H. G., van Dijk, N., van Etten-Jamaludin, F. S., and Wieringa-de Waard, M. W. (2013). The attributes of the clinical trainer as a role model. *Academic Medicine* 88(1): 26–34. doi: 10.1097/acm.0b013e318276d070.

Jones, S. R. (1992). Was there a Hawthorne Effect? *American Journal of Sociology* 98(3): 451–468. doi: 10.1086/230046.

Kenny, N. P., Mann, K. V., and Macleod, H. (2003). Role modeling in physicians' professional formation: Reconsidering an essential but untapped educational strategy. *Academic Medicine* 78(12): 1203–1210. doi: 10.1097/00001888-200312000-00002.

Maheux, B., Beaudoin, C., Berkson, L., Côté, L., Des Marchais, J., and Jean, P. (2000). Medical faculty as humanistic physicians and teachers: The perceptions of students at innovative and traditional medical schools. *Medical Education* 34(8): 630–634. doi: 10.1046/j.1365–2923.2000.00543.x.

Merriam-Webster OnLine (n.d.). S.v. "apprentice." Retrieved from https://www.merriam-webster.com/dictionary/apprentice.

Merriam-Webster OnLine (n.d.). S.v. "role model." Retrieved from https://www.merriam-webster.com/dictionary/role model.

Paice, E., Heard, S., and Moss, F. (2002). How important are role models in making good doctors? *BMJ* 325(7366): 707–710. doi: 10.1136/bmj.325.7366.707.

Passi, V., Johnson, S., Peile, E., Wright, S., Hafferty, F., and Johnson, N. (2013). Doctor role modelling in medical education: BEME Guide no. 27. *Medical Teacher* 35(9): e1422–1436. doi: 10.3109/0142159x.2013.806982.

Ramani, S., Gruppen, L., and Kachur, E. K. (2006). Twelve tips for developing effective mentors. *Medical Teacher* 28(5): 404–408. doi: 10.1080/01421590600825326.

Rose, G. L., Rukstalis, M. R., and Schuckit, M. A. (2005). Informal mentoring between faculty and medical students. *Academic Medicine* 80(4): 344–348. doi: 10.1097/00001888–200504000–00007.

Sachdeva, A. K. (1996). Preceptorship, mentorship, and the adult learner in medical and health sciences education. *Journal of Cancer Education* 11(3): 131–136.

Swanwick, T. (2005). Informal learning in postgraduate medical education: From cognitivism to "culturism." *Medical Education* 39(8): 859–865. doi: 10.1111/j.1365–2929.2005.02224.x.

Swick, H. M., Szenas, P., Danoff, D., and Whitcomb, M. E. (1999). Teaching professionalism in undergraduate medical education. *JAMA* 282(9): 830–832. doi: 10.1001/jama.282.9.830.

Wear, D., Aultman, J. M., Zarconi, J., and Varley, J. D. (2009). Derogatory and cynical humour directed towards patients: Views of residents and attending doctors. *Medical Education* 43(1): 34–41. doi: 10.1111/j.1365–2923.2008.03171.x.

Wright, S., Wong, A., and Newill, C. (1997). The impact of role models on medical students. *Journal of General Internal Medicine* 12(1): 53–56. doi: 10.1007/s11606–006–0007–1.

Wright, S. M., and Carrese, J. A. (2001). Which values do attending physicians try to pass on to house officers? *Medical Education* 35(10): 941–945. doi: 10.1046/j.1365–2923.2001.01018.x.

Wright, S. M., and Carrese, J. A. (2002). Excellence in role modelling: Insight and perspectives from the pros. CMAJ: *Canadian Medical Association Journal* 167(6): 638–643.

Wright, S. M., Kern, D. E., Kolodner, K., Howard, D. M., and Brancati, F. L. (1998). Attributes of excellent attending-physician role models. *New England Journal of Medicine* 339(27): 1986–1993. doi: 10.1056/nejm199812313392706.

13

Teaching and Learning Empathy

ASHLEIGH WRIGHT, JEFFREY BUDD, AND REBECCA R. PAULY[1]

Medicus enim nihil aliud est quam animi consolatio—A doctor is nothing
more than consolation for the spirit.

Petronius

In this chapter we provide a review of literature on the benefits of empathy,
along with challenges and reasons for a decline in empathy over time. We
describe curricular strategies and empathy interventions. Additionally, challenges to empathy in the era of electronic health records (EHR), as an emerging issue, are discussed and tips for role-modeling EHR use for learners are
provided.

Objectives

Define empathy and discuss its importance in patient care.
Describe reasons for the decline in empathy.
Describe methods to teach empathy.
Discuss the impact of electronic health records (EHR) on empathy.

James, a third-year medical student rotating on an inpatient internal medicine service, is excited to present his new patient, Sarah, who was admitted the previous evening with complaints of abdominal pain and nausea.
James has concerns that Sarah's anxiety is contributing to her repeated
hospitalizations for pain. The team, however, is convinced that Sarah is
fabricating her symptoms; she previously had a comprehensive workup,

---

1   Ashleigh Wright, M.D., University of Florida College of Medicine, Gainesville, FL.
Jeffrey Budd, M.D., University of Florida College of Medicine, Gainesville, FL.
Rebecca R. Pauly, M.D., F.A.C.P., University of Missouri–Kansas City School of Medicine,
Kansas City, MO.

which failed to show any underlying pathology. She was on their service for three weeks and discharged two days ago. The team audibly groans at the news of her readmission. A new attending, Dr. Smith, joins the team that morning for rounds. The team presents Sarah as a "difficult patient." Dr. Smith explains to the team that it is important to get to the root of the patient's complaints prior to discharge. She enters Sarah's hospital room, identifies herself, and explains her role on the team while sitting down at the patient's bedside. Sarah relates her complaints about failure to diagnose her abdominal pain despite her repeated hospitalizations. Dr. Smith holds her hand, looks her directly in her eyes and says, "I cannot promise you that I will find a solution to your current complaints, but I commit to you that I will listen to you and do my best to help you as much as I possibly can."

After rounds, Dr. Smith congratulates James for his attention to the patient, and they discuss the complex relationship of anxiety symptoms, abdominal pain, and nausea. Upon returning later to the bedside, Dr. Smith asks Sarah why she thinks she has abdominal pain. The conversation gradually transitions to Sarah discussing her friend's diagnosis of pancreatic cancer at an early age. The friend recently died. Sarah was not only fearful of having pancreatic cancer herself, but she also had lost her greatest confidant. She felt she was now alone in the world. After taking the time to address the psychosocial aspects of Sarah's well-being, the team was eventually able to address her anxiety regarding a possible cancer diagnosis. They also provided her with the mental health support needed to deal with the grief of her friend's passing. Feeling that she had been heard, Sarah was satisfied with her evaluation and treatment, and the team arranged for follow-up appointments with a psychiatrist and psychologist. She went home and has not required rehospitalization. James called her a month later, and she reports she is feeling much better.

At the end of his rotation, James took the opportunity to reflect on his inpatient experience. He stated, "Dr. Smith was my first positive physician role model, and I say this having several physicians in my family. I am accustomed to seeing very intelligent physicians dismiss patients' complaints, and I was starting to reconsider my choice to be a doctor. Dr. Smith showed me how an empathetic and thoughtful approach to direct patient care was one of the best diagnostic and therapeutic tools available—even more so than labs and advanced imaging, in my patient's case."

Clinical empathy is a critical component of the good bedside manner that patients seek in their physician. The word "empathy" was coined in the early 20th century, combining Greek "em," meaning "in," and "pathos," meaning "feeling." This combination was an attempt to translate the German psychological term "Einfuhlung," or "feeling-in" (Lanzoni 2015). Clinical empathy is a blend of emotion, cognition, and behavior as a response to patient experiences (Larson and Yao 2005). The primary focus of the health professional is a selfless concern for the patient, with a goal and willingness to help that person (Neumann et al. 2009).

Conceptual Framework

The importance of empathy

Patients and health professionals

Empathy has demonstrated benefits for both health professionals and patients. Health professionals with a warm bedside manner are more effective in patient care (Di Blasi et al. 2001). Furthermore, several studies show that the empathy and quality of the patient–health professional relationship have a positive effect on health care outcomes (Kaptchuk et al. 2008; Kelley et al. 2014; Price et al. 2006). In addition, adherence to treatment recommendations is greatest when patients perceive empathy in their health professional (Kim et al. 2004). Moreover, empathetic interviewing skills promote greater patient disclosure (Maguire et al. 1996). Not surprisingly, patient satisfaction is also greater with perceived empathy (Kim et al. 2004; Menendez et al. 2016). Health professionals' own personal well-being also correlates with empathy (Seo et al. 2016; Shanafelt et al. 2005). More perspective taking and empathic concern may also be protective against burnout in general practice (Lamothe et al. 2014).

Moreover, there are financial implications of empathic medical care. Increasingly, patient satisfaction scores, which are influenced by empathy, determine a portion of reimbursement. More than 70 percent of hospitals and health networks factor satisfaction scores into health professionals' compensation (Boodman 2015). Beyond reimbursement and compensation, poor communication has an overall economic impact in patient care (Thorne et al. 2005). Among primary care health professionals, malpractice claims are inversely related to patient communication and empathy (Levinson et al. 1997).

Learners

Emphasis on empathy is particularly important during a health professional's training. Learners with higher empathy scores show greater clinical competence. In some studies, female learners score higher than their male counterparts do in empathy, suggesting that women may render more empathetic care (Hojat et al. 2002; Thomas et al. 2007). Predictably, empathy scores do not correlate with performance on the Medical College Admission Test (MCAT) or steps 1 and 2 of the U.S. Medical Licensing Examinations (USMLE). Researchers have suggested a correlation between the capacities for empathy and understanding of one's own prejudices and biases, highlighting the importance of not neglecting the learner's paradigms, prejudices, and contextual situations (Pedersen 2010).

Empathy during training

The course of empathy

Research results vary regarding the impact of training on empathy in medical education. Several studies show a decline of empathy during medical school and residency (Chen et al. 2007; Crandall et al. 1993; Feudtner et al. 1994; Hojat et al. 2004; Neumann et al. 2011; Newton 2010; Nunes et al. 2011; Woloschuk et al. 2004). Conversely, other researchers note no significant change in empathy over time (Mangione et al. 2002; Roff 2015). Recent research reexamining the evidence from previous studies shows a "weak decline" in empathy rather than a strong decline, as well as noting a measurement and interpretation error that may explain the decline (Colliver et al. 2010). However, a number of researchers have refuted these claims and issued clarifications about their methodologies and data interpretation (Hojat et al. 2010; Newton 2010; Sherman and Cramer 2010; Mangione et al. 2002; Roff 2015). Overall, most agree that, during medical education, empathy is stunted.

Causes for a decline

Despite controversy regarding the extent of decline in empathy from the beginning to the end of training, studies show key time periods where the decline occurs. Empathetic responses decline as early as the first year of medical school, possibly due to the newly found, rigorous challenges of training (Nunes et al. 2011). In the clinical years of medical school, where students have patient contact, empathy also decreases (Chen et al. 2007; Neumann et al. 2011). During this time, first-time exposure to the realities of illness, death, and suffering may overwhelm learners (Neumann et al. 2011). Lastly, studies have noted a decline in empathy during internship related to impaired sleep, geographic relocation, and the challenges of patient care (Bellini et al. 2002; Rosen et al. 2006).

The nature of biomedical training focusing solely on biomedical information may lead to the neglect of the patient's views, emotions, and life events. These limitations impact not only medical students but also practicing health professionals (Pedersen 2010). Pedersen (2010) notes that medical schools are "accountable for the effects and side effects" of influences on physicians' empathy, and are "in a position to make appropriate changes" (p. 596).

Distress as a key factor for decline in empathy

Encountering callous or inconsiderate behavior results in stress and anxiety, which in turn decreases the ability to empathize (Bellini et al. 2002; Neumann et al. 2011; Shanafelt et al. 2005; Stratton et al. 2008; Thomas et al. 2007). Detrimentally, stress may lead to emotional detachment and a focus on the more concrete, mechanical aspects of care (Neumann et al. 2011). An underlying emphasis on technical competence and objectivity in training rather than compassion and humanism may also contribute to stress, anxiety, and burnout (Coulehan and Williams 2001). In addition, pressure to complete patient-care tasks, and the high volume of material to learn throughout training, can interfere with the ability to remain in touch with groups that provide social support, including family and friends. This social isolation negatively influences empathy (Hojat et al. 2002). Mistreatment by supervisors as well as a lack of role models can also contribute to overall distress and loss of empathy (Feudtner et al. 1994; Silver and Glicken 1990). Lastly, researchers note a decline in emotional intelligence and empathy across medical education, particularly regarding the degree to which learners notice and think about their feelings (Stratton et al. 2008). Unfortunately, the virtues of humanism emphasized in the medical school admissions process are not emphasized or nurtured in medical training (Stratton et al. 2008).

Challenges to empathy

Traditionally, a good bedside manner and empathy are not core aspects of health care (Boodman 2015; Halpern 2003). As discussed earlier, the stress and anxiety secondary to demanding work environments, heavy clinical workload, and cynicism with little emphasis attached to empathy are some of the obstacles that health professionals face daily (Larson and Yao 2005). Although empathy may actually increase efficiency by setting the tone for trust, health professionals often believe that listening to patients requires additional effort that results in anxiety (Halpern 2003). In cases where there may be tension in doctor-patient relationships, health professionals may fail to recognize not only the patient's emotional needs, but also their own negative emotions (Halpern 2003). Some health professionals overestimate their demonstrated empathy (Block et al. 2013), while others simply lack the needed interpersonal skills to read other people (Boodman 2015). Finally, while residents who score higher on well-being scales also score higher on empathy scales (Shanafelt et al. 2005), programs may not provide training in the needed skills and attitudes for producing well-rounded physicians (Clark 2001).

Teaching Empathy

Many consider empathy an art form that is not achievable simply through explicit teaching and mimicking; rather, it develops through the long-term observation of other health professionals and patients explicitly demonstrating empathy. Thus, learning empathy is a slow immersion process in which education programs take an active role in training and developing empathy, and in creating a culture that values empathy and treatment (Larson and Yao 2005). Empathy training must consider the significance of learners' social and historical background, and the impacts that these may have on empathy (Pedersen 2010). Additionally, the formal, informal, and hidden curricula all influence development and promotion of clinical empathy, which curriculum planning needs to address (Neumann et al. 2009). Although researchers have described attitudes and behaviors that are consistent with providing empathetic humanistic care, there is no clear guidance on how to teach these skills (Weissmann et al. 2006). Role modeling by multiple clinical teachers is one of the most important factors influencing the learner's ability to demonstrate compassion and empathy (Branch et al. 2001). While learners often express hope that they will encounter fine role models, they do not actively seek them out; instead, they wait for role models to appear as dictated by clinical assignments (Weissmann et al. 2006). Clinical teachers identified as role models are highly aware of the significance of their day-to-day actions and identify self-reflection as one of the main techniques they use to refine their teaching strategy. One teacher noted, "Formation of residents is a main part of what we do, and residents are influenced by staff behavior. Each encounter with the patient or family or staff is important. We have to be very careful about how we speak to a patient and about a patient." (Weissmann et al. 2006, p. 664).

Teaching empathy at the bedside

Clinician teachers recognized for excellence in humanistic care role-model implicit and explicit behaviors (Weissmann et al. 2006). First, they pay attention to nonverbal behaviors, including tone of voice, pace, and time taken to rearrange the room in a patient-centered position. Second, they demonstrate respect by asking about patient preferences in treatment and negotiating with patients in a kind and tolerant manner. Third, they try to build a personal connection by commenting on patient effects (photographs, slippers, or other items the patients may have with them) and discussing issues unrelated to the patients' medical care (hobbies, interests, pets). Fourth, they elicit and address the patients' emotional responses to illness, responding empathetically to expressions of fear, worry, grief, or anger regarding illness or medical care. Finally, they take the time to debrief after emotional patient encounters, explicitly letting members of the team know that it is acceptable and normal for health professionals to feel emotions and that it is important to reflect on specific issues that may affect their relationships with patients, including countertransference.

Using seminal events

In the clinical setting, events can shape the values and attitudes of team members. These seminal events can teach invaluable lessons, but by their very nature they are unlikely to occur frequently or for everyone during training. Teachers can use their experience to create miniature seminal events, using emotional events, such as breaking bad news, to involve and provoke learners to provide solutions to difficult problems. This technique leads to a sense of accomplishment and lifelong lessons for learners (Branch et al. 2001). Branch et al. recommend asking the following questions when taking advantage of a teaching moment, be it a seminal event or a simple daily occurrence:

How can I foster participation in this activity by multiple learners?
How can I foster a safe environment for students and residents to bring up their own concerns and prior experiences?
How can I create opportunities for practice, feedback, and discussion?
How can I maximize reflection by learners during this activity?

The hidden curriculum and negative role modeling

While the formal curriculum (actual course of study) places emphasis on the development of empathy, the informal curriculum (unplanned instruction, such as hallway interactions) and the hidden curriculum (ideological and subliminal messages of both the formal and informal curriculum) play a recognized role in the development of learners and health professionals. Studies associate inadequate role modeling in the informal and hidden curriculum with the overall decline of empathy during medical training (Neumann et al. 2011). Negative role modeling, where learners see health professionals displaying disrespect and a lack of compassionate care, can produce unprofessional behavior and ethical erosion during clinical training. If students are exposed to negative role modeling, the hidden curriculum has the potential to undermine the objectives of professionalism, ethics, and the art of medicine (Weissmann et al. 2006). Coaching role models to counter the hidden curriculum by overtly demonstrating the importance of compassionate care can play an important role in the development of learners. Further details about role modeling are provided in the chapter on role modeling in this book.

Empathy training interventions

A recent systematic review described educational interventions used in undergraduate medical education that directly teach clinical empathy (Batt-Rawden et al. 2013). These interventions include: patient narrative;

creative art, writing, and drama; communication skills training; problem-based learning; interpersonal skills training; patient interviewing; experiential learning; and empathy intervention. For example, creative writing, blogging, and discussing poetry and short stories help learners appreciate the patient's point of view. In fact, blogging during a clerkship, followed by debriefing, prevented a decline in empathy during the third year of medical school (Rosenthal et al. 2011). Reflective writing, including composing essays from the patients' points of view or reflecting on personal experiences of illness, also positively impact empathy scores (Dasgupta and Charon 2004; Shapiro et al. 2006).

Drama interventions that focus on coaching students "how to act-in-role" enhance empathy (Lim et al. 2011). Dramatized student portrayals of the challenges of aging, followed by small-group discussion, led to non-sustained increases in empathy (Van Winkle et al. 2012). Interventions in communication skills training address the cognitive aspect of empathy and lead to improvement in empathy scales. Activities include role playing followed by coaching on verbal and nonverbal empathetic responses (Bayne 2011; Norfolk et al. 2007; Fernández-Olano et al. 2008). Interpersonal skills training, where a lecture is followed by role playing that is recorded and analyzed by participants, led to significantly increased empathy scores on postintervention testing (Tiuraniemi et al. 2011). In contrast, problem-based learning that explored medical scenarios from different points of view did not significantly improve empathetic actions by health professionals (Karaoğlu and Seker 2011). While not always statistically significant, multiple studies suggest that interviewing chronically ill patients for their individual perspectives leads to increases in empathy. Interestingly, the impact of these interviews may be influenced by gender and personal background (Kommalage 2011; Mullen et al. 2010; Shapiro et al. 2009; Yuen et al. 2006).

Experiential learning is a powerful technique in teaching empathy. In a randomized controlled trial, while students participated in a medical interview, researchers exposed them to auditory hallucinations, allowing participants to experience symptoms of psychiatric disease (Bunn and Terpstra 2009). Another study exposed learners to losses of vision, hearing, manual dexterity, mobility, and other challenges that occur with aging (Varkey et al. 2006). The immersive nature of these programs seems to be important, as both of these studies reported a significant increase in empathy.

Some programs direct residents and fellows to receive formal empathy training. One example, in which residents and fellows participated in three 60-minute empathy-training modules, led to improvement in perception of empathy by patients as compared to a control group (Desmon 2013). Some companies also offer online courses designed to improve the relationship between patients and health professionals. "Empathetics" is a series of online courses with this goal. A 2011 study showed that health professionals who took the course inspired greater trust in their patients than those who did not (Boodman 2015). Empathy courses generally focus on self-monitoring to reduce defensiveness, improve listening skills, and recognize the role of facial expression and body language. Interactive computerized empathy training for oncologists led to increased use of sympathetic statements and more empathetic responses to negative emotions (Tulsky et al. 2011). Oncologists can manage patient distress by recognizing and empathizing with patients' concerns, leading to increased satisfaction, adherence to treatment, and ultimately quality of life. Tulsky et al. noted that, compared with oncologists who did not participate in the empathy training, patients of intervention oncologists reported greater trust in their physicians (Tulsky et al. 2011). Other formal empathy training can include using standardized patient questionnaires to provide feedback regarding use of patient-friendly language; discovering the patient's agenda; body language training; and interacting with the electronic health record (EHR) (Boodman 2015). Health professionals exhibiting low interpersonal skills who received feedback in a nonthreatening environment showed significantly increased scores at six-month follow-up (Mercer and Reynolds 2002).

The most effective way to increase empathy is to create a comprehensive curriculum targeted exclusively to enhancing empathy that utilizes multiple teaching modalities. Bayne (2011) developed a successful program where facilitators:

Discussed empathy decline.
Worked with learners to develop strategies to overcome barriers to empathy.
Utilized communication skills training and role play.

Using the emotional labor framework

Management and organizational research describe the need in professions like flight attendants and bill collectors to develop an understanding of "emotional labor" to manage the organization's emotional culture (Larson and Yao 2005). "Emotional labor" is the process of regulating experienced and displayed emotions to present the professionally desired image during interpersonal interactions at work. Two methods of acting are inherent to emotional labor. "Surface acting" involves only modifying the emotional display—that is, facial expressions, voice, or posture. In "deep acting," individuals try to change their internal emotional state—that is, the perception of the situation—so they can modify their automatic emotional reactions to the situation at hand and their subsequent expressions. Empathy training interventions use the construct of emotional labor. Studies also use this construct as an organizational tool to explore health professional–patient outcomes.

Impact of the EHR

The implementation of the EHR in clinical settings has changed the dynamics of the health professional–patient relationship. Learners train to use the EHR from a technical standpoint, but often neglect the dynamic between the health professional, the patient, and the computer. The computer has the potential to cause physicians to lose rapport with patients. "Informational flooding" secondary to the increasing use of technology after 2000 has led to an "emotional anesthesia" that suppresses our emotions (Neumann et al. 2011). Although some express concerns about the potential for the EHR to overload the relationship between health professionals and patients, one study concluded that the use of EHR on a laptop appeared to improve the ability of first-year residents to communicate with patients compared to the use of a paper chart (Taft et al. 2014). Researchers noted a statistically significant improvement in asking about patients' understanding of the problem, framing information using the patients' perspective, and exploring the acceptability of the treatment plan. The use of the EHR has not led to a decrease in patient satisfaction, although some patients may feel confused about certain behaviors, such as the health professional looking at the computer monitor without explanation (Als 1997). The addition of exam-room computers did not alter the health professional's baseline patient-centered behaviors (Frankel et al. 2005). Those with good behaviors before the computer maintained those behaviors after the computer. Similarly, those with poor baseline behaviors maintained poor behaviors after the computer. For health professionals who need to improve patient-care skills while using the EHR, one strategy is to divide the encounter into patient- and computer-focused stages clearly demarcated by changes in body language and focus of gaze (Duke et al. 2013). By minimizing screen gaze, stopping typing, and turning to the patient, health professionals can display clinical empathy. Learners, by observing such actions, will improve their skills in the setting of role modeling in a one-on-one style of education (Duke et al. 2013). Thus, with minor modifications to the standard methods utilized for imparting skills in bedside manner, health professionals can continue to display empathy in the setting of an EHR.

Tips for role-modeling EHR use for learners

Greeting—Prior to interacting with the patient, have the learner review the patient's EHR. This preparation allows the learner to spend time introducing him- or herself and interacting with the patient before turning to the computer. Also, spatially organize the exam room to optimize good communication.

Set agenda—Inform the patient that you are using an EHR, and verbalize when shifting back to the computer.

Open interview—Avoid interrupting the patient, and use nonverbal skills as you would in a setting where the EHR is not present.

Build the relationship—Maintain visual and verbal contact with the patient as you type in the EHR.

Educate the patient—Assess the patient's literacy while sharing screen information.

Final Thoughts

The clinical case at the start of the chapter highlights the hidden curriculum that de-emphasizes empathy—that is, when the members of the admitting team audibly groan on hearing that Sarah is readmitted and present her to the attending as a "difficult patient." It illustrates the role an attending physician plays in setting the tone for the team. In this case, Dr.

Smith sat down at the patient's bedside, made eye contact, and was able to elicit and address the patient's emotional responses to illness. Furthermore, she held the patient's hand while explaining the management plan, clearly role-modeling empathy for the team.

Key take-home points about empathy

Clinical empathy is an ability to understand a patient's point of view, communicate that understanding, and act in a therapeutic way with that understanding.

Empathy has demonstrated benefits for both patients and caregivers in the form of improved health outcomes, decreased health professional burnout, greater patient satisfaction, and lower risk of malpractice suits.

The decline in empathy during training is multifactorial.

Challenges to empathy outside of training include demanding work environments, heavy workloads, cynicism, and the apparent low importance attached to it.

Effective teaching by role modeling includes exhibiting nonverbal behaviors, demonstrating respect for the patient, building a personal connection with the patient, and addressing the emotional response of the patient.

Empathy courses generally focus on self-monitoring, listening skills, and body language.

Implementation of the EHR has changed health professional-patient interaction. Techniques to role-model when using the EHR include greeting, setting an agenda, open interviewing, building a relationship, and educating the patient.

Questions for Future Research

Empathy declines during training, and increased empathetic behaviors lead to improved patient care. Therefore, demonstrating a method to prevent the empathy decline would be valuable. Can comprehensive dedicated empathy training in medical school and residency prevent the observed decline in empathy?

Research demonstrates that there are short-term gains in empathy following focused training, but no long-term studies have examined the impact of empathy skills training on sustained improvement in empathetic behavior. Can training sustain empathy long-term?

Role modeling plays a significant role in development of both clinical skills and empathy for many levels of learners. Specific empathy training for faculty can also help improve individual empathetic behaviors. Organizations such as the Arnold P. Gold Humanism Honor Society promote the importance of clinical empathy. However, no studies have specifically assessed the impact of faculty development in role modeling on medical student and resident empathy skills. Does training faculty in role modeling improve medical student and resident empathy?

References

Als, A. B. (1997). The desk-top computer as a magic box: Patterns of behaviour connected with the desk-top computer; GPs' and patients' perceptions. *Family Practice* 14(1): 17–23. doi: 10.1093/fampra/14.1.17.

Batt-Rawden, S. A., Chisolm, M. S., Anton, B., and Flickinger, T. E. (2013). Teaching empathy to medical students: An updated, systematic review. *Academic Medicine* 88(8): 1171–1177. doi: 10.1097/acm.0b013e318299f3e3.

Bayne, H. B. (2011). Training medical students in empathic communication: An updated, systematic review. *Journal for Specialists in Group Work* 36(4): 316–329. doi: 10.1080/01933922.2011.613899.

Bellini, L. M., Baime, M., and Shea, J. A. (2002). Variation of mood and empathy during internship. *JAMA* 287(23): 3143–3146. doi: 10.1001/jama.287.23.3143.

Block, L., Hutzler, L., Habicht, R., Wu, A. W., Desai, S. V., Novello Silva, K., . . . Feldman, L. (2013). Do internal medicine interns practice etiquette-based communication? A critical look at the inpatient encounter. *Journal of Hospital Medicine* 8(11): 631–634. doi: 10.1002/jhm.2092.

Boodman, S. (2015), How to teach doctors empathy. *Atlantic* (March 15).

Branch, W. T., Jr., Kern, D., Haidet, P., Weissmann, P., Gracey, C. F., Mitchell, G., and Inui, T. (2001). The patient-physician relationship. Teaching the human dimensions of care in clinical settings. *JAMA* 286(9): 1067–1074. doi: 10.1001/jama.286.9.1067.

Bunn, W., and Terpstra, J. (2009). Cultivating empathy for the mentally ill using simulated auditory hallucinations. *Academic Psychiatry* 33(6): 457–460. doi: 10.1176/appi.ap.33.6.457.

Chen, D., Lew, R., Hershman, W., and Orlander, J. (2007). A cross-sectional measurement of medical student empathy. *Journal of General Internal Medicine* 22(10): 1434–1438. doi: 10.1007/s11606-007-0298-x.

Clark, P. A. (2001). What residents are not learning: Observations in an NICU. *Academic Medicine* 76(5): 419–424. doi: 10.1097/00001888-200105000-00008.

Colliver, J. A., Conlee, M. J., Verhulst, S. J., and Dorsey, J. K. (2010). Reports of the decline of empathy during medical education are greatly exaggerated: A reexamination of the research. *Academic Medicine* 85(4): 588–593. doi: 10.1097/acm.0b013e3181d281dc.

Coulehan, J., and Williams, P. C. (2001). Vanquishing virtue: The impact of medical education. *Academic Medicine* 76(6): 598–605. doi: 10.1097/00001888-200106000-00008.

Crandall, S. J., Volk, R. J., and Loemker, V. (1993). Medical students' attitudes toward providing care for the underserved. Are we training socially responsible physicians? *JAMA* 269(19): 2519–2523. doi: 10.1001/jama.1993.03500190063036.

Dasgupta, S., and Charon, R. (2004). Personal illness narratives: Using reflective writing to teach empathy. *Academic Medicine* 79(4): 351–356. doi: 10.1097/00001888-200404000-00013.

Desmon, S. (2013). 5 ways new doctors fail at bedside manner. *Futurity* (October 28). Retrieved from http://www.futurity.org/5-ways-doctors-bedside-manners/.

Di Blasi, Z., Harkness, E., Ernst, E., Georgiou, A., and Kleijnen, J. (2001). Influence of context effects on health outcomes: A systematic review. *Lancet* 357(9258): 757–762. doi: 10.1016/s0140-6736(00)04169-6.

Duke, P., Frankel, R. M., and Reis, S. (2013). How to integrate the electronic health record and patient-centered communication into the medical visit: A skills-based approach. *Teaching and Learning in Medicine* 25(4): 358–365. doi: 10.1080/10401334.2013.827981.

Fernández-Olano, C., Montoya-Fernández, J., and Salinas-Sánchez, A. S. (2008). Impact of clinical interview training on the empathy level of medical students and medical residents. *Medical Teacher* 30(3): 322–324. doi: 10.1080/01421590701802299.

Feudtner, C., Christakis, D. A., and Christakis, N. A. (1994). Do clinical clerks suffer ethical erosion? Students' perceptions of their ethical environment and personal development. *Academic Medicine* 69(8): 670–679. doi: 10.1097/00001888-199408000-00017.

Frankel, R., Altschuler, A., George, S., Kinsman, J., Jimison, H., Robertson, N. R., and Hsu, J. (2005). Effects of exam-room computing on clinician-patient communication: A longitudinal qualitative study. *Journal of General Internal Medicine* 20(8): 677–682. doi: 10.1111/j.1525-1497.2005.0163.x.

Halpern, J. (2003). What is clinical empathy? *Journal of General Internal Medicine,* 18(8): 670–674. doi: 10.1046/j.1525-1497.2003.21017.x.

Hojat, M., Gonnella, J. S., Mangione, S., Nasca, T. J., Veloski, J. J., Erdmann, J. B., . . . Magee, M. (2002). Empathy in medical students as related to academic performance, clinical competence and gender. *Medical Education* 36(6): 522–527. doi: 10.1046/j.1365-2923.2002.01234.x.

Hojat, M., Mangione, S., Nasca, T. J., Rattner, S., Erdmann, J. B., Gonnella, J. S., and Magee, M. (2004). An empirical study of decline in empathy in medical school. *Medical Education* 38(9): 934–941. doi: 10.1111/j.1365-2929.2004.01911.x.

Hojat, M., Gonnella, J. S., and Veloski, J. (2010). Rebuttals to critics of studies of the decline of empathy. *Academic Medicine* 85(12): 1812; author reply 1813–1814. doi: 10.1097/acm.0b013e3181fa3576.

Kaptchuk, T. J., Kelley, J. M., Conboy, L. A., Davis, R. B., Kerr, C. E., Jacobson, E. E., . . . Lembo, A. J. (2008). Components of placebo effect: Randomised controlled trial in patients with irritable bowel syndrome. *BMJ* 336(7651): 999–1003. doi: 10.1136/bmj.39524.439618.25.

Karaoğlu, N., Seker, M. (2011). Looking for winds of change with a PBL scenario about communication and empathy. *Healthmed* 5(3): 515–521.

Kelley, J. M., Kraft-Todd, G., Schapira, L., Kossowsky, J., and Riess, H. (2014). The influence of the patient-clinician relationship on healthcare outcomes: A systematic review and meta-analysis of randomized controlled trials. *PLoS ONE* 9(4). doi: 10.1371/journal.pone.0094207.

Kim, S. S., Kaplowitz, S., and Johnston, M. V. (2004). The effects of physician empathy on patient satisfaction and compliance. *Evaluation and the Health Professions* 27(3): 237–251. doi: 10.1177/0163278704267037.

Kommalage, M. (2011). Using videos to introduce clinical material: Effects on empathy. *Medical Education* 45(5): 514–515. doi: 10.1111/j.1365-2923.2011.03951.x.

Lamothe, M., Boujut, E., Zenasni, F., and Sultan, S. (2014). To be or not to be empathic: The combined role of empathic concern and perspective taking in understanding burnout in general practice. *BMC Family Practice* 15(1). doi: 10.1186/1471-2296-15-15.

Lanzoni, S. (2015). A short history of empathy. *Atlantic* (October 15).

Larson, E. B., and Yao, X. (2005). Clinical empathy as emotional labor in the patient-physician relationship. *JAMA* 293(9): 1100–1106. doi: 10.1001/jama.293.9.1100.

Levinson, W., Roter, D. L., Mullooly, J. P., Dull, V. T., and Frankel, R. M. (1997). Physician-patient communication. The relationship with malpractice claims among primary care physicians and surgeons. *JAMA* 277(7): 553–559. doi: 10.1001/jama.277.7.553.

Lim, B. T., Moriarty, H., and Huthwaite, M. (2011). "Being-in-role": A teaching innovation to enhance empathic communication skills in medical students. *Medical Teacher* 33(12). doi: 10.3109/0142159x.2011.611193.

Maguire, P., Faulkner, A., Booth, K., Elliott, C., and Hillier, V. (1996). Helping cancer patients disclose their concerns. *European Journal of Cancer* 32A(1): 78–81. doi: 10.1016/0959-8049(95)00527-7.

Mangione, S., Kane, G. C., Caruso, J. W., Gonnella, J. S., Nasca, T. J., and Hojat, M. (2002). Assessment of empathy in different years of internal medicine training. *Medical Teacher* 24(4): 370–373. doi: 10.1080/01421590220145725.

Mercer, S. W., and Reynolds, W. J. (2002). Empathy and quality of care. *British Journal of General Practice* 52(Suppl.):, S9–12.

Menendez, M. E., Chen, N. C., Mudgal, C. S., Jupiter, J. B., and Ring, D. (2015). Physician empathy as a driver of hand surgery patient satisfaction. *Journal of Hand Surgery* 40(9). doi: 10.1016/j.jhsa.2015.06.105.

Mullen, K., Nicolson, M., and Cotton, P. (2010). Improving medical students' attitudes towards the chronic sick: A role for social science research. *BMC Medical Education* 10(1). doi: 10.1186/1472-6920-10-84.

Neumann, M., Bensing, J., Mercer, S., Ernstmann, N., Ommen, O., and Pfaff, H. (2009). Analyzing the "nature" and "specific effectiveness" of clinical empathy: A theoretical overview and contribution towards a theory-based research agenda. *Patient Education and Counseling* 74(3): 339–346. doi: 10.1016/j.pec.2008.11.013.

Neumann, M., Edelhäuser, F., Tauschel, D., Fischer, M. R., Wirtz, M., Woopen, C., . . . Scheffer, C. (2011). Empathy decline and its reasons: A systematic review of studies with medical students and residents. *Academic Medicine* 86(8): 996–1009. doi: 10.1097/acm.0b013e318221e615.

Newton, B. W. (2010). Rebuttals to critics of studies of the decline of empathy. *Academic Medicine* 85(12): 1812–1813; author reply 1813–1814. doi: 10.1097/acm.0b013e3181fa36e7.

Norfolk, T., Birdi, K., and Walsh, D. (2007). The role of empathy in establishing rapport in the consultation: A new model. *Medical Education* 41(7): 690–697. doi: 10.1111 /j.1365-2923.2007.02789.x.

Nunes, P., Williams, S., Sa, B., and Stevenson, K. (2011). A study of empathy decline in students from five health disciplines during their first year of training. *International Journal of Medical Education* 2, 12–17. doi: 10.5116/ijme.4d47.ddb0.

Pedersen, R. (2010). Empathy development in medical education—a critical review. *Medical Teacher* 32(7): 593–600. doi: 10.3109/01421590903544702.

Price, S., Mercer, S. W., and Macpherson, H. (2006). Practitioner empathy, patient enablement and health outcomes: A prospective study of acupuncture patients. *Patient Education and Counseling* 63(1–2): 239–245. doi: 10.1016/j.pec.2005.11.006.

Roff, S. (2015). Reconsidering the "decline" of medical student empathy as reported in studies using the Jefferson Scale of Physician Empathy-Student version (JSPE-S). *Medical Teacher* 37(8): 783–786. doi: 10.3109/0142159x.2015.1009022.

Rosen, I. M., Gimotty, P. A., Shea, J. A., and Bellini, L. M. (2006). Evolution of sleep quantity, sleep deprivation, mood disturbances, empathy, and burnout among interns. *Academic Medicine* 81(1): 82–85. doi: 10.1097/00001888-200601000-00020.

Rosenthal, S., Howard, B., Schlussel, Y. R., Herrigel, D., Smolarz, B. G., Gable, B., . . . Kaufman, M. (2011). Humanism at heart: Preserving empathy in third-year medical students. *Academic Medicine* 86(3): 350–358. doi: 10.1097/acm.0b013e318209897f.

Seo, J. W., Park, K. H., Park, H. Y., Sun, K. H., Park, S. Y., Kim, T. H., . . . Cho, J. (2016). Empathy and quality of life in Korean emergency physicians. *Journal of the Korean Society of Emergency Medicine* 27(2).

Shanafelt, T. D., West, C., Zhao, X., Novotny, P., Kolars, J., Habermann, T., and Sloan, J. (2005). Relationship between increased personal well-being and enhanced empathy among internal medicine residents. *Journal of General Internal Medicine* 20(7): 559–564. doi: 10.1007/s11606-005-0102-8.

Shapiro, J., Rucker, L., Boker, J., and Lie, D. (2006). Point-of-view writing: A method for increasing medical students' empathy, identification and expression of emotion, and insight. *Education for Health: Change in Learning and Practice* 19(1): 96–105. doi: 10.1080/13576280500534776.

Shapiro, S. M., Lancee, W. J., and Richards-Bentley, C. M. (2009). Evaluation of a communication skills program for first-year medical students at the University of Toronto. *BMC Medical Education* 9(1). doi: 10.1186/1472-6920-9-11.

Sherman, J. J., and Cramer, A. P. (2010). Rebuttals to Critics of studies of the decline of empathy. *Academic Medicine* 85(12): 1813; author reply 1813–1814. doi: 10.1097/acm.0b013e3181fa3877.

Silver, H. K., and Glicken, A. D. (1990). Medical student abuse. Incidence, severity, and significance. *JAMA* 263(4): 527–532. doi: 10.1001/jama.263.4.527.

Stratton, T. D., Saunders, J. A., and Elam, C. L. (2008). Changes in medical students' emotional intelligence: An exploratory study. *Teaching and Learning in Medicine* 20(3): 279–284. doi: 10.1080/10401330802199625.

Taft, T., Lenert, L., Sakaguchi, F., Stoddard, G., and Milne, C. (2014). Effects of electronic health record use on the exam room communication skills of resident physicians: A randomized within-subjects study. *Journal of the American Medical Informatics Association* 22(1): 192–198. doi: 10.1136/amiajnl-2014-002871.

Thomas, M. R., Dyrbye, L. N., Huntington, J. L., Lawson, K. L., Novotny, P. J., Sloan, J. A., and Shanafelt, T. D. (2007). How do distress and well-being relate to medical student empathy? A multicenter study. *Journal of General Internal Medicine* 22(2): 177–183. doi: 10.1007/s11606-006-0039-6.

Thorne, S. E., Bultz, B. D., and Baile, W. F., and SCRN Communication Team (2005). Is there a cost to poor communication in cancer care? A critical review of the literature. *Psycho-Oncology* 14(10): 875–884; discussion 885–886. doi: 10.1002/pon.947.

Tiuraniemi, J., Läärä, R., Kyrö, T., and Lindeman, S. (2011). Medical and psychology students' self-assessed communication skills: A pilot study. *Patient Education and Counseling* 83(2): 152–157. doi: 10.1016/j.pec.2010.05.013.

Tulsky, J. A., Arnold, R. M., Alexander, S. C., Olsen, M. K., Jeffreys, A. S., Rodriguez, K. L., . . . Pollak, K. I. (2011). Enhancing communication between oncologists and patients with a computer-based training program: A randomized trial. *Annals of Internal Medicine* 155(9): 593–601. doi: 10.7326/0003-4819-155-9-201111010-00007.

Van Winkle, L. J., Bjork, B. C., Chandar, N., Cornell, S., Fjortoft, N., Green, J. M., . . . Burdick, P. (2012). Interprofessional Workshop to Improve Mutual Understanding between Pharmacy and Medical Students. *American Journal of Pharmaceutical Education* 76(8): 150. doi: 10.5688/ajpe768150.

Varkey, P., Chutka, D. S., and Lesnick, T. G. (2006). The aging game: Improving medical students' attitudes toward caring for the elderly. *Journal of the American Medical Directors Association* 7(4): 224–229. doi: 10.1016/j.jamda.2005.07.009.

Weissmann, P. F., Branch, W. T., Gracey, C. F., Haidet, P., and Frankel, R. M. (2006). Role modeling humanistic behavior: Learning bedside manner from the experts. *Academic Medicine* 81(7): 661–667. doi: 10.1097/01.acm.0000232423.81299.fe.

Woloschuk, W., Harasym, P. H., and Temple, W. (2004). Attitude change during medical school: A cohort study. *Medical Education* 38(5): 522–534. doi: 10.1046/j.1365-2929.2004.01820.x.

Yuen, J. K., Breckman, R., Adelman, R. D., Capello, C. F., Lofaso, V., and Reid, M. C. (2006). Reflections of medical students on visiting chronically ill older patients in the home. *Journal of the American Geriatrics Society* 54(11): 1778–1783. doi: 10.1111/j.1532-5415.2006.00918.x.

Appendix. Preventing Burnout and Promoting Resiliency

The Coach Approach

Option 1

- *Step 1: Be a Mirror*—best used if residents have not quite "owned" the situation yet and you are trying to help them find a way forward

  Start by asking a question, following a statement of where things "seem to be":

  "It sounds like your knowledge base and performance have been excellent, but you are getting poor 360 evaluations on high-stress rotations. Tell me what this year has been like for you. Is this the kind of doctor you envisioned yourself being when you graduated from medical school?"

- *Step 2: Coach by Numbers (a.k.a. Best Possible Self)*

  Help Residents explore the big steps and baby steps for improvement by identifying the 10 out of 10 vision and how to move forward.

  Ask the resident to think about an upcoming challenge or something they want to work on. Have them articulate how it would look if it was perfect (a "10 out of 10") and they had achieved that goal/met that challenge. Then, ask them to describe how they currently are doing in that area on a scale of 1–10 (1—not at all close; 10—epitome of success), and how they can go up 1/2 point in the next 6 weeks. The goal is NOT to give advice, but to prompt self-exploration of the goal.

  1) If you were a 10 out of 10 on this, what would it look like?
  2) How would you rate yourself now?
  3) What could you do over the next six weeks to raise yourself half of one point?

Option 2: PERMA—Positive Emotion, Engagement, Relationships, Meaning, Accomplishment

Explore the pathways to well-being and happiness. Are they on the right path? Is their work fulfilling?

To explore those pathways, ask the following questions:

- *P—Positive emotion*—What did you feel best about this year? Was there a peak experience?
- *E—Engagement*—What was the most compelling and interesting experience this year?
- *R—Relationships*—Describe a rewarding experience with a patient, colleague, friend or family.
- *M—Meaning*—Looking back over the year, when did your work really matter to someone?
- *A—Accomplishment*—What accomplishment(s) are you most proud of?

Courtesy of Kerri Palamara, M.D., Massachusetts General Hospital, and Carol Kauffman, Ph.D., Institute of Coaching (permission granted by Dr. Palamara via email communication, March 27, 2016).

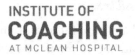
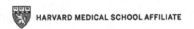

INSTITUTE OF
COACHING
AT MCLEAN HOSPITAL

HARVARD MEDICAL SCHOOL AFFILIATE

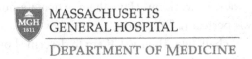

MASSACHUSETTS
GENERAL HOSPITAL

DEPARTMENT OF MEDICINE

Index

Zareen Zaidi is associate professor of medicine and associate chief for faculty development in the Division of General Internal Medicine within the Department of Medicine at the University of Florida. She is director of longitudinal portfolios for the UF College of Medicine and director of scholarship for the Department of Medicine. She has completed her Ph.D. in medical education from Maastricht University, Netherlands. Her research interests include undergraduate medical education, workplace-based assessment, portfolios, qualitative research, critical theory, critical discourse analysis, and cultural competency.

Eric I. Rosenberg is professor and chief of the Division of General Internal Medicine in the UF Department of Medicine. He also serves as associate chief medical officer for UF Health Shands Hospitals. He has collaborated with health sciences center faculty on studies of medication safety as well as development of patient safety curricula. He is regularly invited to provide instruction on patient safety, quality improvement, and preoperative assessment for CME.

Rebecca J. Beyth is professor within the Division of General Internal Medicine at the University of Florida. She also serves as a physician at UF Health Internal Medicine and the Malcom Randall VA Medical Center. She is the author of 90 peer-reviewed publications and 11 book chapters. Her research interests and expertise are in chronic diseases, health promotion, risk stratification, evidence-based medicine, quality improvement, and improving the processes of care.

Printed in the United States
By Bookmasters